Live to be 100 without medicines

Prevention Guide for Optimal

HEALTH

A health guide based on proper nutrition

JULIAN ARAMBURO

Printed in the United States of America

Disclaimer

The nutrition and health advice in this book is based only on the training, education and research of the author. Because each person's body is different and reacts differently to certain foods and medications, the author and publisher encourage the reader to check with a qualified medical practitioner or certified nutritionist before implementing any changes to the diet or life style.
There is always some risk involved in the nature of this subject; therefore, the author and publisher are not responsible for any adverse effects or consequences resulting from the use of any of the suggestions in this book. Please remember that it is perfectly okay to seek a second or third opinion on any diagnosis or advice.

Contact me at my personal email at jaramburo67@gmail.com

Branding and Marketing by www.commva.com

ISBN: 1515175456
ISBN-13: 978-1515175452

LEGAL DISCLAIMER

JULIAN ARAMBURO

DEDICATION

To my beautiful three children and my lovely wife. To my parents who now rest in peace in heaven. To my five sisters and my brother who thanks to God are all still alive and I hope to enjoy their presence, love and company for many years to come. Without my family and close relatives I wouldn't have the happiness I enjoy today. They are the engine that drives me and motivates me to live a healthy life. I also dedicate it to all those who are currently suffering from diseases like Diabetes, Cancer, Heart disease, Alzheimer's and other degenerative diseases. To all of them and the rest of my friends and relatives who I cannot mention because I will need a 300 page book just to cover them all. I thank them for listening to my advice and suggestions to implement healthy life style changes and eating habits. I will continue to outer my discussions on prevention as I know that is the true formula to living healthy, without pain or fear to develop chronic diseases such as cancer, diabetes and others.

Table of contents

Introduction   Page 1
My story   Page 7
Preface   Page 10
Essential ingredients, water   Page 18
Oxygen   Page 24
Exercise   Page 28
Vitamins   Page 33
Vitamin C   Page 45, 95
Juicing   Page 48
Getetically Modified Foods or GMO's   Page 56
FDA approved drugs   Page 60
Statin drugs or Cholesterol medicine   Page 70
Hydrogenated oils or trans fats   Page 79
Omega 6   Page 6, 81
Monosodium Glutamate or MSG   Page 82
High Fructose Corn Syrup or HFCS   Page 88
Artificial colors and flavors   Page 90
Artificial sugars   Page 91
Foods to avoid   Page 92
Essential foods   Page 93
Importance of supplements   Page 94
Diabetes   Page 102
Heart disease   Page 111
Cancer   Page 119
Milk   Page 123
Mammography   Page 127
pH or Potential Hydrogen   Page 132
Alzheimer's disease   Page 138
Obesity   Page 144
Vaccines   Page 161
The miracles of herbs   Page 178
Summary   Page 190
Appendix   Page 193
Recipes   Page 201

ACKNOWLEDGMENTS

Writing this book took me longer than I thought because my goal was to finish it in two years. There are many reasons why I could not achieve that goal but nonetheless it's done and I'm happy that I finally get a chance to share this information with you. I am thankful to God that I can offer my hard work and dedication throughout these years. It has been many nights of little sleep and long hours of review and research. This could not have been achieved without the support of my family. Thanks to my dear wife for helping in one way or another. I Never thought writing a single page would take so much time and effort. Of course it takes so long because the investigation and verification of a particular topic takes a long time to make sure it is correct and the supporting data is accurate. I also want to thank the people who listen to my daily sermon of health through different avenues like family reunions, email and Facebook. When I thought no one was listening or paying attention, I started noticing that gradually my friends and family began to change their lifestyle and to some extend their eating habits. I have received many emails, calls or comments from several people who are grateful for the information I provide to them and because some way or another it has changed their lives and opened their eyes to realize that processed foods are responsible for most of today's health statistics. I feel satisfied when I get those kinds of emails or calls; it gives me great happiness to know that little by little each of those people will be doing their part to transmit that information to other people. I strongly feel that one day large food and pharmaceutical corporations will be forced to change their products to healthier choices. This is actually happening now and I am very happy about it.

I also want to thank my friend Marcos Garcia for helping me edit part of this English version of the book. Thank you Pablo for designing the cover page. Many people contributed to this project which I finally completed and I hope it serves as a guide to educate people of all ages. May God bless you with good health and happiness and please help me change the lives of your friends and family.

INTRODUCTION

Dear reader and friend, I started writing this book primarily for my family and my closest friends; however over time I realized that this book will also serve to educate people to achieve long lasting life free of diseases that are now part of the worst health statistics in the US and the rest of the world. During the last 8 years I've had the fortune to embark in a life changing path of good health. Every person has a story that has changed his or her life or an event that makes them focus on a particular purpose with a certain objective. My purpose (at least for now) is to communicate to all of you what I've learned in the last 8 years on how to live a healthy and long-lasting life completely independent of pharmaceutical drugs.

When I say long-lasting life, I want you to understand that living to be 100 years old (with good health) is not impossible. In Okinawa, Japan and Ville-Cabamba, Ecuador for example, many elderly people have the privilege of being known worldwide and mentioned in many notable publications for their longevity and healthy life style. Many live well over one hundred years of age with good health, thriving and serving in their communities.

According to the many books and scientific articles on health the human body can live a relatively healthy life for 120 years, provided they take care of their body and soul throughout their lives. Many people tell me that today people live more than before; but those statistics include everyone "living" in nursing homes and on life support in hospital beds across the USA and the rest of the world. Believe me there are many of them. Unfortunately many of those elderly people are living with Alzheimer's, dementia and other illnesses that degrade their quality of life. I personally don't call this living since many of those people prefer to be dead than "living" in those conditions. I have visited nursing homes in the United States and I can tell you it is one of the most depressing things I have seeing in my life. Some of them spend most of their days sitting on a wheel chair staring at the wall or focused on a painting on the wall. The smell inside these places is not necessarily the most pleasant and the visitors don't stay inside for too long. What I'm trying to make you understand is the fact that these people are not living to their full potential most likely due to the food choices they made through their entire life or perhaps because the drugs they are taking has turned them into "living" zombies. It is pretty sad if you ask me.

Living with a chronic illness for 10 or 15 years is something very common nowadays and some of these illnesses are classified as terminal; but not all of us have to be part of these statistics. You can change your own destiny by making changes in your eating habits and/or the type of food you eat. You basically need to make a life and death decision when it comes to your diet, exercise and life style. If you don't take action and make changes today, you will most likely be part of these statistics when you get to your 60's or 70's. Some people actually believe that late 60's and early 70's is too old and say things like "why live any older anyway?" well, I believe you should enjoy life way beyond your 90's with good health, why not? Many people in other countries do, so why not you? Why not live to celebrate your 100th birthday and see your great grand kids grow up?

The table below includes the most recent statistics in the United States on the main causes of death as it relates to illnesses and accidents.

No.	Causes of Death	Deaths / Year
1	Heart Disease	611,105
2	Cancer	584,881
3	Respiratory Diseases	149,205
4	Accidents (Unintentional Injuries)	130,557
5	Stroke	128,978
6	Alzheimer's	84,767
7	Diabetes	75,578
8	Influenza, Pneumonia	56,979
9	Nephritis, Nephrosis	47,112
10	Suicide	41,149

CDC data as of 2013

One of the main purposes of this book is to educate you with the necessary tools so you are not part of these tragic statistics. I hope you realize that the human body has the capacity to heal itself and of living many years without suffering with pain or illnesses that deprive you of enjoying a long healthy life. However, you have to help yourself and do your part. Reading this book is only the beginning of your work. To assimilate, embrace and most importantly, take action and implement changes of at least 80% of this information is the other part. To do this you need to make a decision and have the willpower to do it for you and your family. You have the power to avoid living your last days confined in a nursing home or laying on a hospital bed for the rest of your late years. My suggestion is to invest in your health today, so that you don't regret it tomorrow. Unfortunately, we don't appreciate our health until it is too late or until we face a chronic disease like cancer, diabetes or heart disease.

As I mentioned before, everybody has different reasons to write a book or to communicate what has been learned. This book is not the exception. My reason is my family. Unfortunately my dear mother and my father are part of the statistics I mentioned earlier. My mother, Barbara Rita, for example, died from diabetes at the age of 71 (a very young age). My father, Angel, died from lung emphysema at the age of 80. These two ages are young if you ask me. 80 years is a young age if they're lived healthy, without bad habits, a balanced diet and regular exercise. My mother's last 10 years weren't the healthiest by any means. She had many health complications and among other situations, she was subjected to daily insulin injections every morning and evening, which my brother-in-law Jaime administered.

As a result of this disease, she also suffered from high blood pressure, cataracts, aches and pains and symptoms that in several occasions my mother said she preferred to die than to continue with her suffering. In my opinion all these symptoms (outside of her Diabetes) were caused by the drug she was taking for that terrible disease. Later in this book I explain that all pharmaceutical drugs have side effects. These drugs can cause other diseases as well as series reactions to other drugs including death.

Dear reader my biggest desire is to help you find the necessary keys to help you live for many years without having to depend on a wheel chair or prescription medications that can have dangerous side effects. In this book I will also teach you how to read the ingredients of most of the products your family consumes on a daily basis and I explain which ingredients you should eradicate from your diet and which ones to start consuming right away. If you don't think you have the will and cannot take the necessary steps to achieve a long healthy life, at least do it for your children or a loved one who might be suffering and slowly going the path of the statistics mentioned above. Don't make the same mistake that many people make by saying *"I prefer to live 20 years less but eat and drink whatever I please"*. The fact is, you will not only live 20 years less but the last 5 or even 10 years will be so unhealthy and miserable that you will actually prefer to die, as it is the case of the people I mentioned earlier from the assisted living communities. And if you have the unfortunate fate of being diagnosed with Alzheimer's disease, your loved ones will have to take care of you and suffer while you die slowly without knowing what's going on around you.

I hope this book will make you reconsider and understand that we all come to this world to live our full potential and with some kind of purpose in life. What's yours? Mine, at least for now, is probably to reach out to you and to help you understand the importance of prevention through healthy eating. I want you to understand that we dig our own graves with the help of a fork and a knife and the bad habits we make in life.

Approximately 70% of the products we eat are responsible for most of the chronic diseases like cancer, heart disease, diabetes, arthritis and others. The reason is because these products are highly processed and contain a number of ingredients and preservatives that the human body cannot digest, absorb and properly metabolize. If this book changes the way you eat and therefore gives you the health you deserve, then I'll consider that my years of research, reading and writing were not in vain. I hope that when you finish reading this book you are one of those who will join me in my mission to communicate and educate your friends and family and perhaps save their lives.

Remember that eating healthy will allow you to live a healthy productive life free of disease and fear from the flu or a virus floating around you. That's the motto of this book and I trust that you will put aside the unhealthy, cancer causing foods that are making you sick and start implementing better eating habits. The key to living healthy is in eating highly nutritious food, vitamins, minerals from fruits and green vegetables, lots of water and exercise regularly. This will change your life, I guarantee it.

I want to explain one thing about this book. This book is brief and to the point and therefore it should be used as a health guide and not as an encyclopedia. Many of the issues described here can easily take the space of a 400 page book. That's precisely what I wanted to avoid since books over 250 pages end up in an office bookshelf and are never read. I opted for summarizing several topics in a brief book with the hope that you will supplement it with further reading of a particular topic with other books focused on that topic. Also, the publishing house of this book has limits on the number of pages for it to be sold at a reasonable price.

WHY DID I WRITE THIS BOOK?

There are many reasons why I felt compelled to write this book but I'll summarize a few of them here.

I wrote it thinking about my family, friends and everyone that can benefit from this information to live a long healthy life.

Because I want you to know that the death statistics from properly prescribed, FDA approved drugs are horrible and not acceptable and you have options to choose a different path

Because one out of two Americans die of heart disease and one out of three die of cancer. I want you to know how to prevent and potentially cure these and other chronic diseases.

Diabetes is the #7 cause of death in the USA. My beloved mother died of diabetes and I believe the drugs she was taking helped her deteriorate her health and eventually killed her.

I want you to know that prevention based on a good, nutritious diet is the best way to avoid any disease.

Many of the ingredients in most of the processed foods cause the majority of the chronic diseases.

Because you need to know that a balanced diet based on certain fruits and vegetables and free of meats and dairy products can cure almost any disease including diabetes and some types of cancer?

Drugs are not the solution to the problem. Prevention based on good nutrition is perhaps the only solution. Drugs don't cure diseases, they only treat their symptoms.

Opinion – Cancer is preventable and even curable without drugs or radiation if drastic and extreme dietary measures are taken. **JFA**

6

MY STORY

In August 2002 when I was just 34 years old, I experienced one of the worst scares of my life. On a Friday morning at about 8:15 AM, I left my home to go to work. My car was a little old and it decided to die at a red light in the middle of a very busy three lane intersection in West Palm Beach, Florida. Every time the light changed to green, the cars behind me started beeping and changing lanes. I was in a situation where I had to move the car one way or another before someone could hit me. It was the middle of an intense summer with temperatures in the high 90's and very humid. The heat was intense, but I had to push the car to safety. The safest place was about 150 feet away in the parking lot of a supermarket. When I was about 40 feet away from the parking lot, my physical condition did not allow for more, but fortunately a few young Mexican construction workers jumped from a van and helped me push those last 40 feet. *Thank you very much*, I said. Due to the heat and my poor physical condition at the time I started to hyperventilate and I was about to pass out. My limbs felt very weak and started to retract; I started to panic and not knowing what was going on, I thought I was getting a heart attack or something similar. A lady who was passing by saw me and asked me if I needed help; I couldn't respond properly as my speech was hindered by the extreme hyperventilation I was suffering. I eventually passed out and woke up in an ambulance heading to Wellington hospital in Palm Beach County. After a few routine checks and a brief description of what happened, the doctor told me that all the vital signs were normal. The only thing that happened was that due to my poor physical health I started to hyperventilate. Honestly, I never heard that word before. I couldn't believe that I was in such poor fitness condition at only 34 years of age. I was always very active playing soccer, riding my bike, playing racket ball and other sports. I had a GYM membership since I was 16 years old. However, soon after I got married in 1996, my wife got pregnant and our beautiful daughter, Nathalie, was born. My sport life changed dramatically (at least for about 8 years). Approximately seven months later after that episode, I had a similar incident at my house while talking to John, my brother-in-law. We were talking about a few things that were happening to me at the time. Some of them were - The news that my wife was pregnant with our 3rd child after learning that I was losing my job, the death of my father, my 5 month old son fractured his leg and two other minor incidents. Apparently talking about these things caused me a stress level that I couldn't perceive. In the middle of the conversation, I felt a strong chest pain and when I stood up to get a glass of water, I fainted and dropped almost on John's arms. Fortunately, he is a professional fire fighter and a paramedic and after calling 911 he knew what to do until the ambulance arrived. They didn't take me to the hospital that time but the paramedic who assisted me told me the following after checking my blood pressure, pulse and other routine checks - *"You better start exercising and relief your stress or something more serious is going to happen to you"*.

It would've been obvious to have started exercising soon after this incident but that wasn't the case. It wasn't this that made me realize that I had to change my eating habits and start exercising again. It was about two years later when I felt a strong pain on my heart while sitting on my desk at work. One of my arms started feeling numb (I can't remember which one); so I called the doctor's office and the lady on the phone told me to go to the hospital and meet the doctor by the entrance. As you can imagine I sort of panic a little as I thought I was going to have a heart attack. But, how could that be? I was too young to have such symptoms. The nurse and doctor did all the routine checks such as blood pressure, electrocardiogram and others, but everything was kind of normal. At the hospital I was given a stress test on a tread mill but that was also kind of okay. *So, what's going on?* I asked. I was totally confused. The doctor gave me a blood test prescription to check for cholesterol and glucose due to my family history of diabetes. All my confused thoughts became clear when I received a call from the doctor's office (about a week later) to let me know the blood test results. The lipid profile test indicated my total cholesterol was not in the normal range as well as my triglycerides and LDL (bad cholesterol); my HDL or good cholesterol was too low at 34. The glucose level was also a little high which placed me in the pre-diabetic range.

These results were enough evidence that I needed to make a drastic change to my overall health and life style. I should mention that prior to making a drastic change in my diet I used to eat at fast food restaurants almost 5 times a week during lunch time at work and 2-3 times a week for breakfast. I also used to buy Coca-Cola by the cases and drink 2-3 a day. I lost a lot of weight by just not eating the hamburgers and sugary breakfast and removing sodas from my diet. I also gained my energy back. So, I stated eating healthier and exercising again. I knew that the more years will go by the worse my health and the blood test results were going to be. It was then that I started educating myself on how to eat healthy and how the body works when the correct food is ingested VS the wrong foods. I started reading books, magazines and scientific journals on health. The more I read the more I wanted to know about how to reach optimal health and keep the body free of diseases and aches without the need of potentially harmful drugs. I learned to listen to my body better and to know what foods my body didn't agree with and which food gave me energy and vitality. Today, I live a healthy and vigorous life and my blood tests are now in the normal range and they continue to improve each year. I also have the perfect weight for my height. I achieved this without the use of any FDA approved medicines.

Please remember that if you choose to make drastic changes to your diet you must first discuss it with your medical doctor and let him/her know what you would like to do, especially if you are currently taking any prescription medications.

The body is a complex machine and it has millions of molecular, biological and chemical interactions, which make each person different. This difference in body chemistry makes it possible for some people to react different than others when taking a certain medication. Some people may have positive reactions to one drug while others may have very negative reactions that result in death. In this book I will explain what to do to have a balance of all these interactions so the body can use the immune system to heal itself. The body has the ability to heal almost any disease as long as you provide it with the correct food and supplements needed to make it happen. The body is like a car, if you take good care of it by changing the oil, tires and brakes in a preventive way, that car is going to last you a long time. However, if you only change the oil every 30,000 miles and the tires every 100,000 miles, that car will not last more than two or three years, tops. Similarly, your body will work better if you nourish it with the proper nutrients, antioxidants, minerals, vitamins and enzymes needed to create an internal balance, free from disease, toxins and free radicals that constantly attack the immune system.

PREFACE

Not long after the incident that changed my way of eating, I also became interested in reading health publications and how the body works in relationship to the homeostatic balance and the physical, chemical and emotional imbalance. It all started when I had the urge to know the side effects of the medicine, Sopenex, which was prescribed to my son Alejandro. This medicine has more than fifteen side effects, of which Alejandro experienced about five. So I decided to find out about these effects and why it had so many - I consulted medical textbooks and homeopathic books (alternative medicine) and compared the differences between the two. I found that the conventional medicine as we know it today is based on pharmaceuticals and not on prevention of diseases. It focuses in treating a symptom rather than trying to fix the root cause of the disease. I found more answers in the alternative approach to a disease than the conventional methods which have many side effects. It made more sense to me that once a diagnosis is given, that's actually the best time to start asking questions, rather than to stop and prescribe a medicine to treat it. Alternative medicine explains that each person's body has the ability to heal itself if the patient is serious and takes drastic measures such as those that I took a few years ago.

Hippocrates, the ancient Greek physician, is rightfully called "The Father of Western Medicine", favored the use of diet and exercise as cures. He acknowledged and valued the importance of food. He also recognized the diseases that result from poor nutrition. This is now being recognized in modern science today. The biggest issue is trying to make the patient understand that poor nutrition, dehydration and lack of exercise are the main causes of disease. It is very difficult to change the mindset of a person who wants to be magically healed or cured in minutes with the help of a pill.

Among the topics that I present to you here, you will find extensive information about the internal balance, how to get it back and how to keep it.

The majority of the drugs approved by the Food and Drug Administration (FDA), have side effects ranging from minor or moderate, to major and extremely harmful to potential death. According to the Center for Disease Control (CDC) and the death statistics, FDA approved drugs are responsible for more than 100,000 deaths each year, just in the United States of America. Unfortunately, the majority of the doctors don't have the time to explain to their patients (in their 2-5 minute interaction at the doctor's office) that the drugs don't necessarily work for every single person. Every human body reacts differently to medications as I explained earlier. As an example, if a person is prescribed a drug for the flu and that person gets healed the next day in a miraculous way, that doesn't mean that the same drug will work for every patient. All of us will react differently to the same drug. No pharmaceutical company can deny or debate this fact. Through my research I found that a person's ability to cure a disease is heavily influenced by the food that is consumed. On the other hand, if you consistently eat food that lacks the necessary nutrients, vitamins and minerals you need, you could inadvertently be causing the most hated and well known chronic diseases such as diabetes, cancer and heart disease. This is why if you smoke and frequently eat at fast food restaurants, you will be more prone to these illnesses, as well as the "normal" aches and pains that 85% of the population suffers from today. Having said this, do you really want to be part of the death statistics? or do you rather live a healthy and productive life and enjoy it to its full potential until 100 years of age or beyond? It is your choice and only you have the power to make the switch and change your life. No one can do it for you. Do it for you and your love ones, especially your children who will love to see you at their soccer games, graduation or wedding ceremony. Wouldn't you like to see your grand kids grow and play? Of course you would.

Another very important aspect of living healthy is exercise. It is extremely important to understand that eating healthy is not the only answer; you also need to move your body to be healthy. Exercise doesn't have to be hard; you can adapt different routines starting from walking a block or two and then slowly increasing the activity to a mile or beyond. Exercise is recommended outside and preferably in a local park where there are lots of trees to breath pure air and let your mind relax from everyday stress and digital gadgets. Moderate to aerobic exercise can be implemented as you get more into it. I always say, listen to your body and don't overdo it. If your body is telling you to stop or something hurts, Stop! Don't push it. If you do too much too quickly, you may get discouraged due to injury or pain. One of the reasons why aerobic exercise is so beneficial to your health is because it increases heart rate and forces the lungs to inhale more oxygen and exhale more carbon dioxide. This helps the heart work better - remember that the heart is also a muscle and it needs exercise to work better.

While exercising it is best to eat healthy fruits and vegetables, hopefully 100% organic. Why 100% organic? Well, unfortunately in the USA and other industrialized countries, large food companies such as Monsanto and others use pesticides, herbicides, fungicides and genetically modified seeds to help grow conventional fruits and vegetables bigger, faster and resistant to bugs. The problem is that these chemicals are dangerous and have shown in independent scientific studies to cause Parkinson's disease, Leukemia, Nervous system breakdown and endocrine problems. Fruits and vegetables that are 100% organic don't have these issues and should be your first choice for most of these foods.

The Food and Drug Administration of the United States approved the use of the word Organic as follows:

100% Organic – This means that 100% of the ingredients are actually organic and haven't been injected with hormones or antibiotics.

Organic – This means that 95% of the ingredients are organic but 5% have been sprayed with pesticides or contain hormones that facilitate rapid growth.

Made with organic ingredients – It should be noted that only 50% of the ingredients are organic while the rest are artificial and a few products contain genetically modified foods.

After learning about this, imagine then the amount of genetically modified foods that your family consumes in a daily basis. It is believed that 75% to 80% of the products sold in the United States as "food" are highly processed and 80% of these contain genetically modified organisms or GMO's. Later in this book I will explain GMO's in more detail and what the potential negative health effects are. These vary from artificial flavors and colors which cause allergic reactions and other illnesses, to toxic ingredients such as Monosodium Glutamate or MSG which is a known neurotoxin that excites and kills brain cells and affects the nervous system. MSG may also contribute to the generation of cancer cells. I will also include a list of ingredients to avoid so you can prevent many of the known diseases.

In this book you will find information to help you understand the proper balance of fiber, protein and calorie intake. This balance is very important to help the body properly digest and metabolize the foods you eat to covert them to the necessary nutrients, fats, amino-acids and enzymes that your body needs. This helps the organs work more efficiently which in turn help with the pH balance and overall homeostatic balance of the body. When this balance is reduced, the immune system weakens and there is greater chance of getting attacked by external and internal toxins and therefore getting sick with the most common diseases such as the flu or allergies. Toxins are basically poisons that can cause severe illnesses and can be deadly if digested in large quantities. Many of these toxins enter the body via medicines and food as well as through the skin and respiratory system thanks to the contaminated environment. What can we do? It is essential to provide the body with foods high in nutrition and low in calories and sugars that stimulate the internal organs and skin (the largest organ of the human body) so that it can fight these toxins naturally. Remember that the human body has the ability to heal itself. I will also show you how to avoid chronic diseases such as diabetes, cancer and heart disease among others. I also explain which foods are best suited to possibly reverse these diseases.

It should be noted that the medical education in the United States does not always include courses in nutrition and prevention. Medical training emphasizes in the treatment of patients through laboratory products (pharmaceuticals) that often don't provide the advertised effect but rather cause other health problems or secondary diseases which in some cases could be fatal.

This doesn't mean that drugs should always be rejected or avoided; or that doctors should never be consulted. Of course doctors need to be consulted and they are extremely essential to your health. We need them for many different reasons. I actually have a huge respect for doctors (but not for the Medical System). Some examples of when you need to see a doctor or take medications are: If you step on a rusty nail, you must go immediately to a hospital or an emergency center to make sure you are treated with antibiotics to avoid an infection with serious consequences. Also, if you break a leg, the first thing you may want to be prescribed is a strong medication to mitigate the pain and then a specialist (orthopedic doctor in this case) to help you heal that broken bone. Antibiotics are also necessary and essential in certain circumstances and have saved many lives. However, some doctors are prescribing antibiotics to some people who cannot tolerate them or for certain cases that are not justifiable. Antibiotics can cause very serious side effects including food allergies, poor absorption of foods and other serious stomach problems. If you or your children must take antibiotics because of a true bacterial infection, please take probiotics to restore the good bacteria in your gut also known as intestinal flora.

Another very important point is that not all doctors are created equal. Some of them are great doctors and some of them are not so great in my opinion. As noted by Mike Adams from Naturalnews.com in one of his many articles, in 1952 Dr. Chester Southam injected cancer cells to several prisoners at the Ohio State Prison as part of an experimental program sponsored by the National Institute of Health or NIH. These people didn't know they were being injected with cancer cells, much less that they were part of an experiment. In 1962, the same doctor injected 22 elderly patients of the Jewish hospital in Brooklyn, New York, with cancer cells to discover the secret of how healthy bodies fight the invasion of malignant cells. The hospital administration tried to cover up this experiment but in the end this doctor was put on probation for one year by the board of doctors in New York. You would think that this doctor should've lost his license for this wrong doing and put in jail for a long time. Well, guess what happened to this doctor two years later? Dr. Southam was named vice president of the American Cancer Society. Amazing right? This is why I don't donate to this organization. Believe me this is just one of thousands of cases of corruption that are written in the sad history of certain doctors and institutions in this country. For more history on the corruption of the medical system visit naturalnews.com. Unfortunately there are a few doctors who after several years of practice have lost the human sensitivity part of being a doctor and only see dollar signs when treating their patients. Remember that they are also making a living and they have to pay for their cars, homes, medical education debts and medical malpractice insurance which are very high.

Now, if you are a doctor, please don't take this the wrong way. I have a lot of respect for doctors, as they are well prepared and study many years to offer their knowledge for the good of humanity. That's something to admire and be proud of. I am sure that most of the doctors studied many years of their life because they have passion for their career and because they want to heal their patients. Such is the case of Dr. Monica Florez who is a pediatrician in Palm Beach County, Florida who cares for her young patients and speaks with their parents of the importance of good nutrition and prevention. Outside her office, she is also in contact with her patients who keep her busy even during her time off. An example she gave me one day when we were talking about the health of her patients is that she takes the time to speak with parents about their children's health from a preventive point of view based on proper diet. The problem she has is the fact that insurance companies don't pay her any money for that preventive discussion with the parents. Why? Because that discussion is not part of an approved charge code in the insurance books. I explain this in more detail in the following pages.

I also want to mention Doctor Javier Prettelt (Palm Beach County) who takes the time to talk with his patients and ask about their history and some family background before entering into the diagnosis and possible treatment of his patients. Some of you may be asking, but isn't that what doctors are supposed to do? The problem is that doctors in the United States have to examine many patients each day to cover all costs associated with the office, employees and the high cost of malpractice insurance. That is why the average time a patient interaction with a doctor (in USA) is 7-10 minutes, but many doctors only have time to listen to their patients for about 20-30 seconds before being interrupted by a nurse or another doctor. That causes medical errors that can be fatal in some cases, especially in hospital emergency rooms.

Now, the biggest problem is that health insurance companies are really the "Monarch" of the medical system and they only pay a doctor when a diagnosis code is submitted; without this code the doctor cannot charge for the patient's visit and all the doctor can charge is the co-payment, which is relatively low. Many people don't know that if the doctor spends 20 minutes telling the patient or the patient's parents to eat healthy, to not drink sodas, to lose weight, to drink more water, etc. insurance companies pay zero money to that doctor. This is unfair because prevention based on good nutrition is the first weapon a doctor has to help patients avoid getting sick and keep coming back. What does this mean? Well, in my opinion it means that "health" insurance companies are not interested about prevention or a healthy patient. Remember, these companies exist because of sick people not healthy people. Without sick people, insurance companies make no money so they have no incentive to pay for prevention. People don't understand this so let me explain how HMO's work and why they are the cheapest in the United States. The example below is given in the book "Ultra Prevention" by Doctor Mark Hyman and doctor Mark Liponis.

Example: If you visit the doctor because you are complaining of chest pains and the doctor tells you to take a test, but that test is not included in the insurance charge codes, the HMO will not cover that test until the patient suffers a heart attack. To keep costs down, insurance has a list of approved codes. If a drug or a test is not on that list, as in this example, the insurance will not cover it. It doesn't matter if the doctor tells the insurance that without this test the patient may experience a heart attack. In this case, this doctor is trying to prevent the patient from having a heart attack but the insurance company doesn't recognize the effort of this well intended doctor. The patient is forced to pay thousands of dollars for preventive tests that are not included in the insurance codes. This is why I believe the "Medical System" in the United States should be reformed completely so that we, the people, have better options for disease prevention. Educate yourself and remember that if you don't make a decision to change the way you eat and your lifestyle, you will be part of the death statistics sooner than you may think. We all dream of enjoying our golden years, so why not do it with good health and vitality.

In the following pages I will show you a list of ingredients and suggestions that are essential to everyone, regardless of their health status. These basic ingredients are probably more powerful than conventional medicine and in many cases they have miraculous healing effects. Medical doctors today are slowly accepting the healing values of these and are beginning to inform their patients of the importance to incorporate them. Slowly but surely prevention will be part of the medical system; well, okay that's my hope.

Join me to discover the secrets of good health to live without fear of the worst diseases that continue to add to the death statistics. (Remember that every decision you make in this book should be discussed with your medical doctor).

ESSENTIAL INGREDIENTS

WATER

If you are wondering why I chose water as the first ingredient in this list, well, as most people know, the human body consists of approximately 75% to 80% water. Water is absolutely essential. For this reason the human body needs to hydrate constantly. Water serves not only to hydrate but also to oxygenate, lubricate joints and help the digestive system do its job. Not all water is created equal, however. The water coming into your home, depending on the processing efficiency of the public purification plant, may contain different levels of waste, chemicals and sediments including Chlorine, fluoride, lead and others. Make sure you know and read the report of the quality of your local city water. This is available upon request from any municipal water utilities department. Many experts agree and recommend never to drink water directly from the tap, unless you have a reliable water purification system. The most recommended by experts is Reverse Osmosis System; but if you cannot afford this type, at least use a carbon water filter that removes most chemicals and sediments, that's better than just drinking water without filtration. Zero Water is a brand recommended by some experts. Also, you need to understand that not all bottled waters are the same; some are as bad as tap water. One of the main issues with bottled water is that the plastic releases a chemical called BPA or Bisphenol-A (when heated or frozen) which has been shown to mimic estrogen and other hormones. It is also an endocrine disruptor which is a substance that interferes with the production, secretion, function and elimination of natural hormones. Babies and young children are more sensitive to the effects of BPA. If you buy bottled water I advise you to buy filtered water from natural springs (spring water) in a glass bottle, or even better, purified water with a Reversed Osmosis System; read the label and find out before you buy. Another option may be distilled or boiled water. Water is so important that experts explain that a person should drink half his weight in ounces, daily. For example, if you weigh 120 pounds, you should drink 60 ounces of water each day. Note that sodas and other non-natural beverages are not part of those 60 oz. Below you will find a section that explains the dangers of sodas and other sugary drinks.

A word of caution on water consumption - Drinking water is very important but you need to make sure you are drinking at least 2-3 cups of water enhanced with electrolytes. You can also take electrolyte supplements. You need to do this because when you drink too much water you also go to the restroom more often and every time you urinate you release small amounts of essential minerals the body needs to function properly. The way to tell is by looking at the color of your urine. If it doesn't have a yellowish color and instead is looking kind of clear, you need to replenish your body with electrolytes to compensate for the loss. My recommendation is to make your own electrolyte water by adding lemon juice, cucumber slices, orange slices and a pinch of Himalayan sea salt to your filtered water. There are other recipes that make delicious electrolyte water. Just do a quick Goggle search and presto!

Water in its natural state in rivers, lakes and wells can contain large amounts of bacteria and other organic pollutants, so it must be treated in municipal processing plants to make it suitable for human consumption. During this process of filtration and purification, chlorine and other chemicals are used to "clean" the water and kill disease causing bacteria. But depending on the processing capability of the treatment plant, some bacteria can travel in the water supply along with residues of potentially dangerous chemicals. Again, depending on the person's health and metabolism and the volume of waste in the water, these chemicals can accumulate in the human body and cause serious health damage. Unfiltered water can also cause skin irritation and may contribute to hair loss.

Chlorine, for example, accumulates in the body and can slowly affect the arteries causing injuries to the outside walls. Chlorine can also cause skin rashes and allergies. An injured artery causes plaque buildup that eventually raises blood pressure.
Note that pools with purification systems using chlorine can contribute to the accumulation of this chemical in your body because it can easily get absorbed through the skin.

Fluoride is another chemical used in some city's water treatment plants. It is a very dangerous chemical that accumulates in the body and it is very difficult to remove.

Fluoride is present in many toothpaste brands and is used by dental hygienist as part of the cleaning process.

According to the Environmental Protection Agency or EPA, fluoride is more harmful than lead in parts per million or PPM; however, city drinking water has a higher content of fluoride than lead. Why is this allowed? Many cities adapted this chemical into their water supply a long time ago when fluoride was thought to have amazing benefits for teeth health. This could not be further from the truth. Fluoride can be deadly if accidentally consumed. This is why many of the popular tooth paste brands have a warning statement on the back of the label that reads *"If more than used for brushing is accidentally swallowed, get medical help or contact a poison control center right away."* Watch your little kids when they are brushing their teeth.

My recommendation is that you improve the quality of your own water supply at home by installing a whole house water purification system for you to enjoy healthy water at the shower and the tap. Some of these filtration systems cost between $200 and $5,000 depending on the sophistication level. If you can't afford the most expensive ones, start with a system that you can afford but remember that it is your health that you need to worry about. Any purification system is better than nothing.

Some experts explain that bathing for 20 minutes with no water filtration is equivalent to drinking 4-5 ounces of water directly from the tap. The reason is that the skin pores absorb some of this water especially if you bathe with warm water or warmer than normal. Our pores are capable of absorbing so much that it is now very common to see many popular medications being sold as patches for weight loss, smoking cessation and even as contraceptives. Be careful with those.

The benefits of drinking water are so amazing and here I summarize a few of these. Daily water intake may be one of the most important ingredients for weight loss. How? Water suppresses appetite in a natural way by helping the body to metabolize accumulated fat. The kidneys cannot work properly without the proper water consumption. When water lacks in the system, many of the kidney functions are passed to the liver to keep the body working properly. One of the main functions of the liver is to metabolize fat and convert it to energy, but if the liver has to do some of the kidney functions on top of the 500 other functions that it does; it is obvious that the liver will metabolize less fat and that fat will accumulate in the body which in turn will neutralize weight loss.

Drinking a good amount of water is also very important to help the body eliminate retained water. When you don't drink enough water the body believes it needs to go in survival mode and begins to hold the little bit of liquid it has to survive. This water tends to accumulate in extra-cellular spaces and it shows with swollen feet and hands. Some drugs help with this accumulation of water but do not prevent the body from retaining water again when it needs it. Remember, the body is designed to heal itself and knows what to do when you have a physical or cell deficiency.

One of the most effective ways to help and prevent the body from the accumulation of water is by supplying it with what it needs the most, WATER. This is one of the most effective ways to help the body eliminate retained fluids. Now, if you have a persistent issue related to fluid retention, you may need to change your diet and lower your sodium or salt intake. The easiest way to cleanse the body of excess salt is by drinking large amounts of water. The reason is because the kidneys filter the salt through the urine. Some experts recommend that due to the slow metabolism of obese and overweight people, they have to drink more water than normal. This will help you lose weight because the body dilutes the excess fat to be able to accumulate water needed to metabolize nutrients and filter toxins ingested with some of the foods you eat. Water helps tone muscles and prevents sagging skin that usually occurs after losing weight. It also helps with constipation problems. When the body doesn't have enough water, it absorbs water from other sources; one of those sources is the colon, resulting in constipation.

Something that is very obvious but most people don't know is that water helps to lower blood pressure. Have you ever tried to pass a thick liquid like honey or molasses through a 10 mm hose? It is almost impossible. The same happens when the arteries are clogged with fat or lipids or when there is too much sugar accumulated in the cells. Water helps to dilute sugar and sluggish plaque to increase blood flow. This helps cleanse and oxygenate blood vessels and thus reduce the pressure in the arteries. This point is very important but it is very difficult for some people to understand or implement because they simply don't like to drink water. My advice is to make the water taste better by squeezing a few drops of lemon (which also serves to raise the pH of the water and balance the acidic level of certain foods) and a few slices or wedges of orange. If you add a bit of lemon, please don't add any sugar because this takes away the benefit of drinking water and sugar lowers your pH. More on this in the pH chapter.

Okay but how much water is enough? Most experts suggest that an adult and normal weight person should drink at least 8 glasses of water a day. Obese people should take an extra glass. Other experts suggest drinking about half your weight in ounces as I explained earlier. You can replace one or two glasses of water with 100% juice (homemade without milk) or with enough servings of fruits and vegetables. To give you an idea, an orange contains about 63% water and a cucumber contains approximately 90% water. The juices sold in supermarkets should not be consumed because their glycemic index is higher than normal since they have to be pasteurized to meet FDA guidelines.

If you eat fruits and vegetables every day and at least 6 glasses of water, you will not have to worry about the 8 or 9 glasses of water that experts recommend. Some experts recommend to drink cooler water as it is absorbed into the system more quickly than warm water and can even help to burn more calories. However, I don't recommend drinking cold water after eating a hot meal as cold water can solidify fats, sugars and oils rather quickly and minimize digestion, which can cause heartburn and serious long-term health problems.

The benefits of water can also be seen in better health through better digestion, nutrient absorption, skin hydration, detoxification, etc. Some of the diseases that can be prevented and possibly treated by drinking water include asthma, headaches, migraines, hypertension, arthritis, kidney stones, back pain and ulcers among others.

You may be wondering what the connection is between water and a headache. The brain has a 75% content of water; when the brain detects that there is not enough water in the body, it automatically begins to produce histamines to ration the little water it has. This causes fatigue and what we all know as "headache". These histamines send a message to the body indicating that something is not working well. When we take medicine for headache and anti histamines, analgesics (acetaminophen and ibuprofen) all we are doing is turning off this message and worsening the problem by making it more intense. Taking two glasses of water and resting in a well relaxed way for about 30 minutes is more effective than these drugs without any side effects.

Back pain can also be caused by lack of water since the vertebrate discs have a very high fluid content. These discs are self lubricated as long as there is enough water in the system and a continuous motion (such as exercise). Something amazing and interesting to know is that the discs' fluid support 75% of the body weight while the other 25% of the weight is supported by the outer layer. When a person is overweight or when water levels are minimal (causing dehydration of the discs), the outer layer of the discs have to bear most of the weight causing pain, inflammation or swelling. This is why back pain is most common on people with a sedentary lifestyle or a job that requires long hours of standing or sitting in a routine daily position. To reduce or eliminate back and neck pain as well as knee and other joint aches, I recommend drinking adequate amounts of water every day, take Omega 3 fish oils and make simple movements like bending forward and backwards and stretching to help keep the body lubricated at all times. Walking is also very important because it helps stimulate the lymphatic system which collects and transports all the waste flowing through your blood stream. Remember that a car engine without oil can burn in just minutes; the same thing can happen with the human body if it doesn't have enough water. If I had to choose one thing among all the recommendations in this book I'll advise you to choose drinking plenty of water. Without water, a forest becomes a desert and life would not be possible; so raise your glass of water and say *"To my Health"* Cheers!

OXYGEN

What do I mean by oxygen? Well, remember that the human body is composed of 75% water which is chemically defined by the abbreviation H_2O. These denote two molecules of hydrogen and one molecule of oxygen. The oxygen is transported throughout the body via the blood (the river of life). That's why you feel recharged with a simple sigh of deep breath as those performed by yoga lovers and other meditation techniques. Deep breathing makes the heart expand and rushes blood throughout all parts of the body. Deep breathing also sends enough oxygen to the brain to stay alert. When you provide mouth-to-mouth resuscitation to a person who is not breathing, you are essentially sending oxygen to the brain so he doesn't go into a coma. Deep breathing is extremely important for your health as it helps revitalize cells and strengthen the heart.

Disciplined and continuous exercise is one of the most important things you can do to achieve optimal health. Many people who start an exercise routine, stop doing it for many reasons including work, children and other house related activities. There is an easy way to start over in a very simple way without straining your body. The secret is simply to take deep breaths during the day (2-3 times a day for 30 or 60 seconds each time). If you are exercising or not, focus on the way you breathe. You will notice that you are breathing in a very shallow and superficial way and hence not excelling enough carbon dioxide from your body.

This can cause different types of illnesses such as muscular fatigue or tiredness, mental block and a decrease in tissue function. There are many deep breathing techniques including Yoga, Tai Chi and Qi-Gong. These techniques are so important that there are many resources that explain its effectiveness. Some of these benefits include depression management, anxiety and stress and in some cases can replace psychological treatments and even obesity. A study by doctors showed that most of their patients had an unusually high level of carbon dioxide in their blood but the rest of the blood tests were in normal levels. It was very likely that this was caused by many years of shallow breathing and lack of exercise.

I was very fortunate to practice the movements of Tai Chi with Master Willian Wu in Hong Kong city while visiting the island during one of my trips to China with the company I currently work for. This was an amazing experience and despite the slow movements and not using any weights or machines, the next day I had aches and pains in different parts of the body that I never experienced before; and I usually go to the gym 4-6 times a week. It was truly amazing. Picture below with Master Willian Wu.

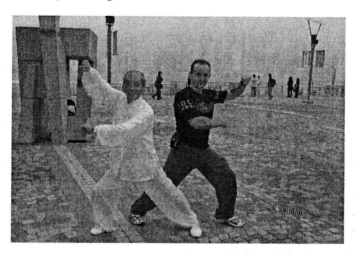

Shallow breathing or chest breathing causes a restriction on the chest and lung tissues, reducing the circulation of oxygen to the tissues of the organs. Deep breathing expands the diaphragm which helps expand the lungs' air pockets and consequently helps pump the lymphatic system. Deep breathing is vital to the lymphatic system in the same way that a pumping heart is to the circulatory system. Cells need oxygen to live and to maintain optimum health the cells need a complex exchange between these two systems. A good circulatory system transports nutrients and an immense amount of oxygen to the capillaries, whereas a healthy lymphatic system is responsible for removing destructive toxins from the bloodstream. Deep breathing is the moderator of this exchange.

Okay so what is the lymphatic system? This is comparable to the sewer system of a large city. Lymphatic vesicles form a drainage system throughout the body. Cells practically swim in an ocean of lymphatic fluid which carries waste from the immune system, including dead white blood cells, plasma and unusable toxins. The lymphatic system is also a defense mechanism of the body. It filters out waste that causes disease; it generates antibodies and also produces white blood cells. The lymphatic system distributes nutrients in the body and drains excess fluids and protein which help prevent swelling of the tissues. This system is made up of a network of tiny vessels that circulate body fluids. These vessels carry excess fluid away from the spaces between tissues and organs.

The negative consequences that result from having a weak lymphatic system are enormous. In some cases they can be fatal because the body doesn't release toxins properly. The most vulnerable people are those who don't engage in regular exercise or don't eat a healthy diet. If you are not breathing deeply and exercising regularly (walking, running, etc.) it is very likely that your lymphatic fluid is not running as well as it should and your body is not in proper balance. As you can imagine, this can cause long term health issues, including weight gain, muscle loss, high blood pressure, fatigue and inflammation.

The good news for you is that deep and proper breathing will help improve the ability to cleanse the lymphatic system. The expansion and contraction of the diaphragm stimulates the lymphatic system and gently massages your internal organs, helping the body rid itself of toxins, leaving more room in the cells for optimal oxygen exchange. Deep breathing not only helps the above systems but also the nervous system and the cardiovascular system.

Oriental cultures have long recognized the importance of breathing to cultivate a positive relationship between body and mind. Asian people practice Yoga, Qi Gong and Tai Chi, which are exercises that combine deep breathing and movement to maintain a more stable central nervous system. This gives us a partial key as to why Asian women report fewer symptoms of menopause, including hot flashes. Several studies in women during menopause show that proper breathing and other relaxation techniques reduce the frequency and severity of hot flashes.

A basic measure of exercise is cardiovascular fitness - which is the amount of oxygen that the heart and lungs deliver to the cells. If you smoke, please stop. Smoking is very damaging to most of the systems in the human body and causes a slow decline in the respiratory and circulatory systems. As I mentioned before, my father died of pulmonary emphysema due to smoking and his ability to breath was reduced dramatically a few months prior to his death.

There are many ways and gadgets to help with proper breathing; one of these is the use of a mini trampoline for 5 minutes per day. This will help pump the lymphatic system more effectively than other products. Another simpler way is to walk 35-45 minutes a day at least 3-4 days a week. As you progress in your exercises, try to increase the frequency and severity. Buy a gym membership near your home and use it at least 3-4 times a week. Invite a friend and set goals to make it more interesting and challenging.

In the next chapters I will explain what to do to lose weight, control your cholesterol and prevent other diseases with just a few changes to your diet and exercise routine. Every doctor and fitness expert will tell you that exercise is as important as drinking water and breathing clean air.

Make time to do some relaxing exercises such as yoga or simply commit to stretching for at least 30 minutes daily. You won't believe the benefits of these simple exercises. This is the foundation of good health and I guarantee you that your heart will thank you. Get your yoga mat and breathe your way to good health.

EXERCISE

Exercise is probably the best way to prevent or cure many diseases that today are needlessly treated with conventional medicine. One of the most notorious and well known universities in the field of medicine in the United States and the world is Mayo Clinic. In its website you can find many health tips and recommendations. In the following link www.mayoclinic.com/health you can find information related to exercise. A good article to read is called "The 7 benefits of regular physical activity". In this article, experts say that in addition to having more energy and possibly live longer, the benefits of exercise extend far more than one can imagine. From preventing chronic health conditions to building self-esteem and confidence and reducing the symptoms of depression; exercise is one of the keys to better health. These benefits are available regardless of age or gender of the person.

In the obesity chapter there is a section by professional personal trainer, exercise science expert and Acute Leukemia survivor, Fabian Valencia, who provides you with great tips on how to lose weight at any age at home without the need of a gym membership or exhausting exercise routines.

The following are 7 great benefits from physical activity according to an article from Mayo Clinic's website

1) Exercise increases well being and overall self esteem. If you need to lower your stress after a hectic day at work, a short trip to the gym or a 30 minute walk will help you calm down. Why is that? Exercise stimulates various brain chemicals, which can leave you happier and more relaxed. Regular exercise will also make you look better and therefore feel better which in turn will increase your self esteem and confidence. Exercise even reduces feelings of depression and anxiety.

2) Exercise fights chronic diseases. If you are concerned about heart disease (and you should because 1 in 2 people die from this disease in the United States each year) or perhaps you want to prevent Osteoporosis; Regular exercise is probably the best thing you can do.

Daily exercise will also help prevent or manage high blood pressure in a more natural way than using prescription drugs. Your cholesterol also benefits. Exercise helps increase good cholesterol (HDL) as well as lower bad cholesterol (LDL). This is very important because this balance helps maintain a smoother blood flow and reduce plaque buildup in the arteries. Another important bonus that comes from daily exercise is the fact that it prevents type II diabetes, osteoporosis and certain types of cancer. Pretty amazing, right?

3) Exercise helps reduce those extra pounds you have accumulated through the years. This is a very basic and obvious side effect of exercise and most people know this but very few people actually do something about it. When you burn calories you lose weight, it's that simple. The harder and longer you exercise the more calories you burn and the faster you lose weight. The only thing I want to warn you about this is to not over do it and to listen to your body and stop when your body tells you. No one knows your body more than yourself so listen up. If you are an active person you don't have to do too much to lose weight. If you want to start slow, use the stairs instead of the elevator whenever possible; take a walk during your break and after each meal; Do some jumping jacks while watching TV, or better yet, turn off your TV and go out for a 45 minute walk. Regular and disciplined exercise is great but daily accumulated activity will also help you burn calories and lose weight.

4) Exercise helps strengthen the heart and lungs. Exercise helps to send oxygen and nutrients to all tissues. In fact, regular exercise helps the cardiovascular system work more efficiently. This is a big deal. When your heart and lungs work better, you will have more energy to do the things you enjoy the most.

5) Exercise promotes better sleep relaxation at bedtime. If you are among the average person who cannot sleep well or take forever to fall asleep, I advise you to start or increase physical activity immediately. A complete and relaxed night can increase your concentration, productivity and well-being. If you have difficulty falling asleep fast, start exercising in the afternoon or at night but try to do it 2 hours prior to going to sleep.

6) Exercise can give you the spark you need to regain the sexual activity that you once had. It you feel too tired to have sex? Or feel very

exhausted after having sex? Exercise may be the solution. Regular exercise can help you feel more energized and looking better, which may have a positive impact on your sex life. Men who exercise regularly have fewer problems in the future when it comes to erectile dysfunction. This is true because exercise increases blood flow in all areas of your body including your privates.

7) Exercise can be fun. If you are disciplined and make time for it, exercise can be fun with your family or friends. Have fun! Exercise doesn't have to be extreme. Dancing, going out with your kids on a bike ride, walk to the park and other activities are perfect occasions to exercise your body and to get out of the daily routine. It also has the nice benefit of getting more connected with your family, especially in the era of smart phones and tablets which are disconnecting families in a very ironic way, don't you think?

In the goal of every person to reach their 65 years of age to retire and enjoy their golden years with their partner, their children and grandchildren, a healthy diet, regular exercise and keeping a healthy weight should also be part of that goal. This will help you live to be one hundred without worrying about dangerous FDA approved drugs but instead living a long healthy life with purpose.

The combination of inactivity and eating what you shouldn't be eating is the second most common cause of preventable death in the United States. Smoking is the first. What does this mean? Regular exercise and good hydration are possibly the most important habits that a human being must undertake since these are the basis and the beginning of the chemical balance that everybody needs. The human body is considered to be in good condition when it is in complete balance. You may be wondering when this balance occurs. The pH level is probably the best way to measure this balance. The pH has a scale from 1 to 14, where 1 represents the most acidic level and can burn a hole through steel and 14 is the most alkaline and extremely pure level. The balance occurs when the body registers a level equivalent to a pH of 7. This balance is very important when trying to prevent and cure cancer and other terminal diseases. Knowing this may very well save your life or your loved ones. I will explain later in more detail the pros and cons of pH and how to measure it at home in a very simple and economical way using pH strips sold at your local pharmacy.

The following are some of the other benefits from regular exercise

- Reduces the risk of premature death
- Reduces the risk of developing or dying from heart disease
- Reduces high blood pressure
- Lowers high cholesterol
- Reduces the risk of developing breast and colon cancer
- Helps prevent Diabetes
- Keeps a normal and healthy body weight
- Aids in the formation and maintenance of healthy muscle tissues
- Helps reduce depression and anxiety
- Provides psychological well being
- Helps to raise the level of performance in sports and at work

How to make exercise a daily habit

- Try to exercise at a specific time

- Sign a contract to yourself dedicating time to take care of your own temple, You.

- Use a calendar and mark the days and time to log physical progress

- Compete with yourself by walking longer or faster each day you go out.

- If you can and have the time, buy a membership at a gym. This is the best way out of the daily routine

- If you suffer from severe inflammatory diseases such as osteoarthritis, I recommend exercising in a pool or in the ocean (watch out for sharks).

Ideal heart rate during exercise

Measuring your heart rate lets you know how hard your heart is working. You can check your heart rate by counting your pulse for 15 seconds and multiplying the result by four.

The below table shows the ideal heart rate when performing any type of aerobic exercise for all ages. When you begin an exercise routine start with the bottom part of the table or 60% as your main goal. As your physical fitness and endurance improves, you can increase your exercise level and increase your heart rate gradually until you reach a level close to 85%.

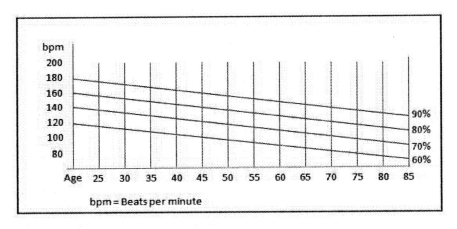

VITAMINS

A lot has been written about vitamins. Some say they are bad, others say they are good; they can cause you harm, they have healing powers; are they synthetic or natural. So many contradictions about this topic and at the end, the consumer doesn't know what to do or who to believe. That's why in this book I have compiled and summarized all the necessary information for you to judge for yourself and make an educated decision when buying vitamins or multi-vitamins. I'll explain which are the best to buy and which to acquire for the best long-term benefit. I will also explain what problems you may face due to deficiencies of certain vitamins. Many of the vitamins that are sold today in pharmacies, supermarkets and retail stores are manufactured in very large laboratories using synthetic ingredients and with very little nutritional value. That's why I always recommend to read the ingredients list and to invest in a good supplement rather than buying the synthetic alternatives.

More than 80 percent of Americans suffer from malnutrition even by government standards. Many people are surprised to hear such statistics because two thirds of the population in the United States is classified as overweight and half of them are obese. Well, I'm not talking about the same malnutrition seen in people of very poor countries in Africa or parts of the Middle East. Such malnutrition is due to lack of protein intake.

I'm talking about a different kind of malnutrition, which is seen in people who eat too much of the wrong foods or foods that have no nutritional value and loaded with calories. Examples of these foods are microwave meals, restaurant food, fast food (junk food), instant foods, packaged foods, refined carbohydrates, etc. etc. In the United States we are proud to say that we have plenty of food to eat and give away. The fact is two thirds are suffering from overweight issues. One of the things many people don't realized is that having those extra pounds doesn't mean they are healthy or well nourished. On the contrary, often being obese or overweight means being sick or malnourished because these people consume foods that are high in calories and deficient in vitamins, proteins and minerals that are essential to the health and daily maintenance of cells and enzymes. Another sad statistic is that 91% of Americans don't get the government recommendation of fruits and vegetables which is five to six servings per day; yet, many experts recommend not only five or six but eight to ten servings a day for optimal health.

The following list constitutes the primary malnutrition of most Americans.

- Antioxidants
- B Complex
- Vitamin D
- Folic acid
- Essential fatty acids
- Minerals such as calcium, magnesium, zinc and selenium

There are approximately 40 essential vitamins, minerals and other organic compounds that the body needs but cannot make by large enough quantities to stay healthy. And it gets even worse as you get older. When these vitamins and minerals work together in an orchestrated way, the body experiences total balance as the millions of cells interact the way they are designed to work to promote optimal health and to promote the growth and reproduction of other cells. Many studies have confirmed that supplementing with vitamins and minerals do much more than just filling the space that every day foods don't fill. Vitamins can prevent or heal the most common health issues like stress, heart problems, cancer and memory loss. You can get some of the nutrients through food but unfortunately the foods consumed in Western countries are highly processed, high in fat, sugar, sodium and refined carbohydrates and are loaded with artificial preservatives to make them last longer on the supermarket shelves. This doesn't allow the organs and digestive system to create enough nutritious enzymes to help the body convert food into protein and nutrients in a natural and effective way. In many occasions the recommended daily allowance or RDA of vitamins is not enough to properly treat or prevent disease. For example, the recommended daily value of vitamin E is 30 IU, but scientists say that one needs 400 IU to 1000 IU daily to reduce the risk of cardiovascular disease. Another example is the recommended value of vitamin C which is 100mg. There are many scientific studies done on this wonderful vitamin where the researchers have given patients up to half their weight in milligrams of vitamin C with amazing results and no side effects. These are just a couple of examples but most if not all the RDA values in vitamins and minerals are way too low according to scientists and doctors.

If you live in Palm Beach County, Florida, before you start taking any supplements, I recommend you to make an appointment with Dr. Leon Camilo Uribe. Doctor Uribe knows the importance of vitamins and other supplements and actually has a machine that measures the level of antioxidants in your body. For a very reasonable cost you will know if the vitamins you are taking are helping you or are just producing expensive urine. He can also recommend you which kind of vitamins to take to raise the level of antioxidants which are extremely important to maintain the internal balance that I mentioned before. That balance is important because the human body is very complex and any imbalance in the chemistry and biology of the organs and overall cellular structure will create havoc and potentially cause allergies that impairs the way the body functions. Allergies are dangerous and can cause many diseases and even death if not treated properly and quickly. Some of the most allergy causing foods that can also cause inflammation and irritation of the intestinal lining are: Wheat and gluten products, dairy, eggs, refines grains, artificial and heavily processed sugars, corn, peanuts, caffeine and processed foods.

Vitamin A

Vitamin A is one of those vitamins that the body needs to perform normal daily functions. This helps in the formation and functioning of healthy teeth, skeletal and soft tissue, mucous membranes and skin. It is also known as retinol because it makes the pigments in the retina of the eye. Retinol is an active form of vitamin A. It is found in animal liver, whole milk and some fortified foods. This vitamin as you know is essential for good vision. Some foods contain antioxidants that protect cells from the eyes of free radicals, which are believed to contribute to certain chronic diseases and play a role in the degenerative processes found in aging. One of the antioxidants that help vision is beta carotene which is kind of dye found in some vegetables.

Vitamin A deficiencies

Vision problems are one of the leading causes of vitamin A deficiency. The person may also be more susceptible to infectious diseases. The best way to acquire the amounts of this vitamin necessary for good health is to eat a balanced diet and take a daily supplement of at least 5,000 IUs. Acute vitamin A poisoning usually occurs when an adult takes several hundred thousand IUs. If large amounts of beta carotene are taken, it can make the skin turn a little yellow or orange, but it returns to its natural color once such consumption is reduced.

Foods that contain Vitamin A

Vitamin A can be obtained from animal sources such as meat and organs, eggs and dairy products. You also get beta carotene from sources such as green vegetables and fruits with strong colors like carrots, red pepper, yellow pepper and green pepper, spinach, kale, beets, squash and sweet potato.

B COMPLEX VITAMINS

These nutrients can protect you from stress by regulating your mood and helps you stay calm. They are also extremely important for the formation of every cell in your body, especially nerve cells. B vitamins - including thiamin (B1), Riboflavin (B2), Niacin (B3), pyridoxine (B6), folic acid (B9), Cobalamin (B12), Biotin and Pantothenic Acid - will help your body generate neurotransmitters, which are brain chemical messengers.
Recent studies led by Dr. David Benton, Ph.D., professor of psychology at the University of Swansea, Wales, shows that vitamin B1 supplements or multi-vitamin supplements containing high potency B complex vitamins can improve your mood. The studied persons taking these supplements reported that they noticed they were more collaborative and tended to agree on unusual situations.
Conversely, if there is a deficiency of these B vitamins it can make you more sensitive to stress and arguments or fights. Studies conducted in the past 50 years have found that low levels of many of the B vitamins are directly connected to emotional problems, including anxiety, nervousness, depression, and even schizophrenia.

How to take them

Start with a B complex that can be purchased in different amounts in milligrams; from 25mg to 75mg. In my case for example, I take 75mg a day on a full stomach.
Two of these B vitamins require a little more attention: Folic acid which must be in the range of 400 to 800 mcg and vitamin B12 between 300 to 500 mcg. Add a little more folic acid and B12 if your multi-vitamins don't

have enough of these. Remember that B vitamins are water soluble. This means they are excreted in the urine and therefore are removed from the body quickly. When you take more than you need, the body accumulates a portion of them in organ tissues, especially the liver, but most are excreted in urine.

B vitamins (B Complex) act as co-enzymes, which are compounds that bind a protein component called Apo-enzyme to form an active enzyme. This enzyme therefore acts as a catalyst in chemical reactions that transfer energy from the food to the entire body. Most B vitamins are categorized as co-enzymes and are essential for facilitating the metabolic processes necessary for life. These vitamins are extremely essential to convert carbohydrates to glucose, which gives us energy to break down fat and protein, which in turn help the proper functioning of the nervous system, muscle tone in the stomach and intestinal tract. Great for healthy skin, hair and eyes.

The B vitamins are important for the proper formation of every cell in your body, especially nerve cells. This is why it is very important that pregnant women take supplements containing B-complex, especially folic acid; and why a deficiency in certain B vitamins is manifested in depressive behavior or intolerable mood.

These vitamins also help produce neural transmitters which are chemical messengers in the brain.

Vitamin B1 (Thiamin)

One of the benefits of this vitamin linked to mental health is the ability to help maintain a controlled temper. It also converts carbohydrates into energy; promotes healthy nerves; helps keep the mind alert; improves the heart's pumping capacity; acts as an antioxidant, which helps protect against the effects of aging, alcohol and cigarettes; aids in the production of hydrochloric acid, which is vital for proper digestion; some studies indicate that this vitamin helps prevent and avoid the increasing effects of Alzheimer's disease; It is also crucial for memory and concentration. Outside of Alzheimer, Thiamin is also prescribed to treat related disorders in the nervous system such as multiple sclerosis, neuritis and Bell's Palsy disease, which is a paralysis of the facial nerve that causes the inability to control facial muscles on the affected side. Another benefit of thiamin is that it can serve as a mosquito repellent, naturally without harmful chemicals. Keep in mind that you will have to take them for at least 4 days before you feel the insect repellent effect.

Vitamin B1 deficiencies

Vitamin B1 deficiency affects the functioning of the gastro-intestinal system, cardiovascular and nervous systems. It can also cause beriberi and Wernicke-Korsakoff syndrome, which is sometimes found in alcoholics. Symptoms of beriberi include loss of appetite, digestive irregularities and a feeling of weakness and numbness in the arms and legs. Other deficiencies of vitamin B1 are depression, memory loss, muscle weakness and stiffness, fatigue, headache, loss of appetite and nausea.
People with the following conditions should consider taking Thiamin (B1) as well as the consumption of fish, and shells fish: Alcoholism, Heart failure, Crohn's disease, Anorexia, Renal Dialysis and Multiple-sclerosis.

Foods that contain vitamin B1

The following foods provide vitamin B1 in a natural way: Organic cereals, oysters, peas, lima beans, peanuts, pistachios, water melon, oats, fish and others foods with less amount of B1. Note that the Thiamin from these foods is lost when foods are cooked at high temperatures. To preserve Thiamin found in foods, cook at low temperatures with less water than normal and try not to overcook them. Steam in order to maintain and preserve the best natural flavor. Other natural sources containing B1 are meat, wheat germ, oranges, brown rice, pasta or noodles.

Vitamin B2 (Riboflavin)

This vitamin works with the other B vitamins to provide the body with energy to metabolize carbohydrates, fats and protein. It also helps in the regeneration of the Glutathione, which is an enzyme that cleans the body from free radicals. This vitamin can also help reduce migraine pain. You can prevent cataracts and plays an important role in the production of hormones to speed up metabolism and helps produce immune cells to fight infections.
The following people are usually deficient in vitamin B2 and probably need extra doses of supplements: Women who are pregnant or breastfeeding, athletes, people who drink heavily and are in extreme stress and those who just had surgery.
This vitamin is best when taken with Manganese, Vitamin C, E and the rest of the complex B.

Vitamin B2 deficiencies

Absolute Riboflavin deficiency is rare but when it occurs, is often related to deficiency of all vitamin B complex deficiency. Usually the deficiency is manifested with problems of the mucous membrane, skin, eyes and blood. Early detection can be clearly seen with peeling and cracking around the mouth. Other deficiencies are noted with dry skin, red eyes and anemia.

If one day you experience the following symptoms please consider taking an extra supplement of vitamin B2 to raise levels of Riboflavin:

• Pain in the mouth
• Swelling of the tongue and lips
• Sensitivity to light
• Itching and dry skin around the mouth, nose, forehead, ears and hair.
• Tremors
• Insomnia

Foods that contain vitamin B2

Birds, fish, fortified organic cereals and grains, broccoli, asparagus, spinach, organic yogurt, organic milk and cheese.

Vitamin B3 (Niacin)

Like all B vitamins Niacin helps metabolize carbohydrates. It is very important for converting calories to energy but also helps with digestive function, promotes normal appetite, lowers cholesterol, helps prevent depression, it is beneficial for arthritis pain, promotes healthy brain and nerve cells, helps the body get rid of toxic chemicals and helps protect the pancreas. It is also believed that niacin helps combat acne, high blood pressure and diarrhea.

There are three forms of vitamin B3: Nicotinic Acid, Niacinamide and Inositol hexaniacinate. Large amounts of nicotinic acid (100mg and 400mg per day) help lower levels of bad cholesterol or LDL and triglycerides, as well as help to raise levels of good or HDL cholesterol. This indicates that vitamin B3 plays an important role in preventing and reversing heart disease. Studies show that this vitamin raises levels of HDL (good) cholesterol more effectively than popular the medicine, Lovastatin. Although Lovastatin helps lower LDL levels better than niacin, niacin also lowers levels of a lipid called Lp(a). According to experts, high levels of this lipid are an additional risk factor for cardiovascular disease.

A note of caution:

High levels of Niacin in the form of nicotinic acid at daily doses greater than 500mg may cause severe side effects such as liver damage, diabetes, gastritis and elevated levels of uric acid. For this reason, scientists and nutrition experts created another form of Niacin called Inositol hexaniacinate which acts as niacin in the form of nicotinic acid but without the side effects. People can take doses up to 3000mg a day of Inositol without risk of liver complications, gastritis or diabetes. Make sure to take this vitamin after eating a meal or you may flush all over your body, especially your face; you may also experience an uncomfortable itching. There is a non-flush form of Niacin so look for this on the package when you shop for this vitamin.

Vitamin B3 deficiencies

A small deficiency of this vitamin can cause side effects such as reducing a person's tolerance to cold as this deficiency lowers metabolism. A severe deficiency of this vitamin can cause serious health problems including a disease called Pellagra, which causes symptoms that include weakness, dermatitis, diarrhea, dementia, sensitivity to light, mental confusion, insomnia and skin lesions.

Foods that contain vitamin B3

Beef liver, tuna, peanuts, salmon, ground beef, peanut butter, cooked potatoes, pasta, mushrooms, barley, mango, almonds, corn and sweet potato.

Vitamin B5 (Pantothenic Acid)

This vitamin is essential for the growth, reproduction and physiological functions because it is found in all cells of the body. Its name comes from the Greek word meaning Pantos which means, in every part. Vitamin B5 is a co-enzyme which like other B vitamins, help with the metabolism of carbohydrates, protein and fat. This vitamin has many features and benefits including: Maintaining a healthy digestive tract, skin and glands; Converting cholesterol to anti-stress hormones and reducing skin allergic reactions in children. It is also known as the stress vitamin. This vitamin can be useful in the treatment of rheumatoid arthritis and may lower cholesterol and triglyceride levels.

Vitamin B5 deficiencies

Some of the problems that can cause a deficiency of this vitamin are respiratory infections, fatigue, headache, hair loss and hair discoloration, mental depression, dizziness, muscle weakness, indigestion, nausea, low blood pressure, neuritis and psychosis.

Foods that contain vitamin B5

The best food sources that contain this vitamin are eggs, beef liver, nuts, soy, peas, mushrooms and wheat germ.

Vitamin B6 (Pyridoxine)

This vitamin is essential for the production and multiplication of red blood cells and anti-bodies needed to fight virus and other diseases. Therefore it is essential to the mucous membrane function, skin and brain chemistry. This vitamin helps to heal depression and helps with issues related to insomnia. But the most important benefit of this vitamin is its association with the treatment of several different illnesses including Autism. The reason is because in several studies, Autism has been connected with the reduction of several neural transmitters that require vitamin B6 to promote a healthy brain function. In numerous studies it has been shown that people with low levels of Pyridoxial-5-Phosphate (a form of B6) in their blood have a five time higher risk of suffering a heart attack than those with normal levels of this vitamin.

Help maintain a balance in sodium and potassium and it uses fat and protein appropriately to control a healthy weight. Finally, it promotes a healthy skin and reduces inflammation of the tissues.

Vitamin B6 deficiencies

As I mentioned before, the lack of sufficient quantities of this vitamin can cause depression and hair loss as well as anemia, arthritis, acne, convulsions in babies, dizziness, nervous system disorders, skin irritation, muscle cramps, overall weakness, urinating issues and learning problems.

Foods that contain vitamin B6

The best sources to get this vitamin outside of supplements are bananas, wheat germ, eggs, meat, melon and green vegetables.

Vitamin B7 (Biotin)

Biotin is a co-enzyme that helps with the metabolism of fatty acids and amino acids. It is necessary for the growth of cells and carbon dioxide transfer. It also helps maintain a regulated blood sugar level. This vitamin is often recommended for strengthening hair and nails. Plays a role in the citric acid cycle, or Krebs, which is a process by which biochemical energy is generated during aerobic breathing. Biotin relieves muscle aches, eczema and dermatitis and also helps combat depression and drowsiness.

Vitamin B7 deficiencies

A deficiency of this vitamin is rare and seldom seen but can result in deterioration of metabolic functions as well as nausea, vomiting, anorexia, paleness, depression, colitis, dry and scaly dermatitis.

Foods that contain vitamin B7

It is found in foods such as liver, egg yolk, mushrooms, some vegetables like cauliflower and potatoes, fruits like bananas, grapes, watermelon, strawberries, yeast, milk, almonds, nuts, fish, chicken and royal jelly. The recommended daily dose is 300 mg.

Vitamin B9 (Folic Acid)

Folic acid is an essential vitamin because it plays a very important role in cell division and the formation of DNA. One of the most important medical discoveries of the 20th century is that when a woman wants to get pregnant or is already pregnant, she must take this vitamin because it can reduce the risk of birth defects associated with neural tube. This tube is tissue in the shape of a cylinder approximately the length of the embryo that eventually forms in the central nervous system. If the tube doesn't close at the top part, the baby is born with a smaller or no brain, resulting in infant death within hours or days after birth. If the tube is not closed at the bottom (in the base of the spinal cord) this can result in paralysis or in many health issues related to the nervous system. Most birth defects occur in the first weeks of getting pregnant when most women don't even realize they are. This is why supplementing with this vitamin is extremely essential before you get pregnant. It is even more essential for women who take birth control pills because one of the side effects of these pills is to reduce levels of folic acid; Unbelievable but true. Several studies show that folic acid provides the best protection three months before conception and during the first three months of pregnancy.

I want to repeat to women the following; because I think it's vital information. One of the side effects of the pill is reduced folic acid levels. If you are a woman please take note of this extremely important B vitamin. This can be considered one of the worst nutritional crimes of the twentieth century. You read it correctly, the association of folic acid and prevention of birth defects is one of the most significant medical discoveries of the twentieth century. This is why I repeated it and want you to help me pass this news to your family and friends. The most unfortunate thing is that this discovery did not make the big news and most people still do not know the benefit and importance of this vitamin. The one thing we have seen in recent years is the addition of this supplement to many cereals and other foods; however, that amount is insignificant and in most cases, this added vitamin is the synthetic form with very little nutritional value.

Folic acid can be used as an analgesic for muscular pains; also helps with the formation of organs and the development of muscles, production of hydrochloric acid, cell formation, helps with digestion, with protein metabolism, with the formation of red blood cells and it helps the nervous system as it makes a protective layer around the nerves protecting them from nerve damage.

Vitamin B9 deficiencies

Some of the deficiencies associated with this vitamin (folic acid) are fatigue, insomnia and loss of appetite and as I said before, can cause birth defects. A recent study says that vitamin B9 deficiency in women who are pregnant, cause an increased risk of conceiving babies who would be more likely to be autistic. People with little folic acid in their diet or supplements may be more prone to certain cancers. Deficiency of this can be manifested through the following symptoms: slowed growth, graying, tachycardia, depression, nausea, fatigue, weakness, low weight, lack of appetite, mouth ulcers and tongue sores.

Foods that contain vitamin B9

The animal kingdom contains low levels but is found in beef liver and chicken liver, organic raw milk and its derivatives. The plant sources are lentils, spinach, cabbage, lettuce, asparagus, wheat germ, bananas, melon, orange and avocado among others. Raw vegetables retain higher levels of this vitamin because cooking and heating reduces or destroys the natural content of folic acid.

Vitamin B12 (Cobalamin)

This vitamin is extremely important to your health because it plays a major role in the formation of red blood cells and in the normal functioning of the brain and nervous system including the spinal cord. This vitamin is water soluble and helps the metabolism of each of the cells of the human body, especially in the synthesis and regulation of DNA. It also aids in the synthesis of fatty acids and the production of energy.

Helps in organic processes including nutrition, digestion, absorption, elimination, respiration, circulation, and temperature regulation. It is essential for the body to absorb iron and prevent anemia. Many doctors consider vitamin B12 as a rejuvenating tonic. Helps restore appetite and energy to patients recovering from a recent operation. It helps children growth and gives them more appetite. This vitamin can also be useful in cases of numbness and tingling in the extremities. Helps detoxification or elimination of cyanide from the body caused by pesticides and other toxins found in the environment.

On the subject of muscle growth, this vitamin helps with the formation of creatine which is essential for muscle energy reserves and protein mass development. This vitamin is sold in several forms. Buy methylcobalamin or hydroxocobalamin. The other form is Cyanocobalamin but it is not recommend because it has been questioned about its safety as cobalamin is processed with small molecule amounts of cyanide to form Cyanocobalamin. This is the cheapest form of this vitamin. If you are taking a multivitamin that has B12 in the form of cyanocobalamin you don't have to stop taking it but I advise you to buy a separate vitamin B12 supplement in the other two forms described above.

Vitamin B12 deficiencies

The deficiency of this vitamin can cause memory loss, disorientation, irritability, hallucinations, loss of reflexes, metal fatigue, insomnia and even depression. It is extremely essential for older people as their B12 levels have been measured in the low ranges and this can cause mental problems. Some doctors supplement with vitamin B12 for people who abuse alcohol, drugs, people with chronic gastritis, with hyperthyroidism, smokers and people who have a poor diet. Like any other vitamin B complex, vitamin B12 should be taken together with the rest of the B complex vitamins because a deficiency of one can cause deficiencies of the other.

Foods that contain vitamin B12

Besides meat and fish, vitamin B12 is found in eggs and all dairy. Adults need at least four or five micrograms of this vitamin daily to reach optimal levels in the body. Remember that every human body is different and therefore the doses are not the same for each person. Educate yourself and read more about this and the rest of the B complex family to maintain a healthy central nervous system.

Vitamin C

This is my favorite vitamin and, in my opinion, everyone should take at least 1000 mg daily. This vitamin has been mentioned in many books not only by doctors and nutritionists but also by Nobel Prize scientists, like Doctor Linus Pauling who is the only one who has won two Nobel Prizes without having to share it with another scientist.

A few of the many books about this wonderful vitamin are: How to live longer and feel better; Cancer and Vitamin C; Vitamin C - The real story; Orthomolecular Medicine; Curing the incurable; Doctor Yourself, etc. Many books and articles have been written about this vitamin and its healing effects. In this book, I can only mention a few of these positive effects and benefits as well as the problems that can arise if this important supplement is ignored.
Massive doses of vitamin C can cure almost everything; as it is explained by doctor Linus Pauling, Dr. Frederick Klenner, Dr. Irwin Stone and Andrew Saul, PhD. What do I mean by massive doses? To answer this we have to start with the doses recommended by the American Medical Association, which suggests a daily dose of only 60mg. This amount is negligible and can be acquired by eating certain foods like oranges, strawberries and others. Many experts agree to use large amounts of this vitamin. For example, Dr. Linus Pauling explains that a person weighing 210 pounds can take up to 35,000mg divided into 17 to 18 doses daily. This amount sounds excessive to most people, but Dr. Klenner used up to 4 times this dose by intravenous injection with amazing results. People with high sensitivity to citrus fruits, tomatoes, sour cranberries or blueberries cannot take the acidic type of vitamin C. These people should take Calcium Ascorbate which is gentler to the stomach, and the digestive system absorbs it more effectively.
Vitamin C or ascorbic acid as it is most commonly known is an extremely essential nutrient to humans and animals in general. The presence of this vitamin is required for a number of metabolic reactions in all animals and plants and is created internally by almost all organisms, except humans a d

primates. Its deficiency causes scurvy in humans, hence the name of ascorbic acid. Ascorbate is an antioxidant, since it protects the body against oxidation and is a cofactor in several vital enzymatic reactions. The animals that can produce its own vitamin C are able to do so by converting glucose into vitamin C; but as I said above, humans do not have this capability because the enzyme that processes this synthesis is absent.

Vitamin C is a potent antioxidant that works to reduce the oxidative stress in the body.

This vitamin acts as an electron donor to 8 different enzymes:

• Three enzymes that help in the hydroxylation of collagen. Thus vitamin C becomes an essential nutrient for the maintenance and development of scar tissue, blood vessels and cartilage.

• Two enzymes are necessary for the synthesis of carnitine. This is essential for the transport of fatty acids into mitochondria to generate ATP which is the main fuel that gives you energy.

• The remaining three enzymes have roles in dopamine, hormonal function and metabolism to help in the food absorption process.

The biological tissues that accumulate more than 100 times the blood levels of vitamin C are: The adrenal glands, pituitary gland, thymus gland and the retina.

Those with 10 to 50 times the concentration present in the plasma include the brain, spleen, lung, testis, lymph nodes, mucous of the small intestine, leukocytes, pancreas, kidney and salivary glands.

Vitamin C helps with the development of teeth and gums, bones, cartilage, iron absorption, growth and repair of normal connective tissue, collagen production, metabolism of fats and wound healing.

White blood cells contain 20-80 times more vitamin C than blood plasma, and it strengthens cyto-toxic capacity of white blood cells.

Vitamin C is essential for the development and maintenance of all tissues and the body in general, and therefore their consumption is extremely essential to your health.

Vitamin C has many uses:

Prevents premature aging, protects connective tissues. It facilitates the absorption of other vitamins and minerals. It serves as an antioxidant and it is one of the reasons it prevents degenerative diseases such as atherosclerosis, cancer, Alzheimer's disease and heart disease among others. Some time ago when cold medicines were not as popular or had not been released, vitamin C was used by doctors as a preventative method to boost the immune system and cure certain diseases. Scientist, Linus Pauling, said that high doses of vitamin C have anti-cancer powers. Later I will give more benefits of this miracle vitamin.

Glutathione

Glutathione is an extremely important substance produced by the liver. This is also found in fruits, vegetables and some meats. This substance is as important as vitamin C and is known as the mother of all antioxidants. Many people have never heard of this substance but it is one of the most important in preventing cancer, dementia, heart disease and aging of cells. It is being used for the treatment of autism and Alzheimer's.

As explained earlier, the body produces this molecule but you have to do your part for the liver to produce it since poor diet, drugs, toxins, stress, pollution, age and radiation reduce the ability to make it. The liver like any organ in your body has some capability to work effectively. This capability is reduced when the liver is overloaded by high levels of oxidative stress, free radicals and disproportionate and long term consumption of medicine.

JUICING

This is a very important topic and recommended by many experts and doctors of natural and homeopathic medicine. I want to clarify that the juices I discuss and emphasize in this book are not the ones you buy in your local supermarket which are bottled and nicely sealed. Those juices don't have the same nutritional value as a homemade juice because the FDA requires those juices to be pasteurized. Pasteurization kills all the benefits of the small amount of juice in that bottle. It also increases the glycemic index of the product which causes the pancreas to excrete more insulin than needed. In short, do not drink bottled juices from supermarkets and limit yourself to make your own juices. In this chapter I explain which fruits and vegetables are important for your health and which combination to use to get more energy, fiber and even to detoxify your body. On this subject you can write an entire book as it is very important for overall health, but I will give you a summary in this part of the book.

Those who don't eat fruits or vegetables in the proper amounts are missing the amazing benefits that these promote in the body. Some of these benefits are - to strengthen, purify, revitalize, detoxify, rejuvenate and rebuild the cells in every corner of the body. One of the easiest ways to absorb the necessary amount of fruits and vegetables is by juicing them using a reliable juice extractor. When you juice your own fruits and vegetables you know that the juice you are drinking is pure and free of preservatives, heavy processing or is not pasteurized like all bottled juices found in supermarkets. You also know that this wonderful and miraculous liquid goes directly into the blood stream and your body doesn't have to work too hard to absorb it, digest it and properly metabolize it. Another important benefit of homemade juice is that you know that the fruits and vegetables that you use are fresh and have a high content of vitamins, minerals and essential nutrients that facilitate their absorption, especially if they are organic. There are several clinics in the United States using juice extraction (among other things) as part of a healthy program to cure degenerative diseases such as diabetes, heart disease and even cancer in some cases. One of these centers is the Gerson Institute in California. This institute is truly amazing when it comes to healthy living. This is one of the few institutes that are actually curing diseases and have done it for many years. One of the ironic things about the medical system in the USA is that the FDA doesn't allow this kind of institutes to make any claims related to curing cancer or other degenerative diseases because they are doing it without the use of FDA-approved drugs. The sad thing is that, in my opinion, FDA approved drugs used to treat cancer are extremely dangerous and barbaric; such is the case of chemotherapy and radiation. These institutes are curing diseases like cancer with non traditional methods like juicing, highly nutritious foods, coffee enema and other completely natural therapies without any side effects. It is unfortunate to hear when friends and family are diagnosed with cancer and the only treatment that oncologists have to offer are chemotherapy and radiation. Those who don't know about these barbaric methods don't realize the damage until it is too late. Most of the patients that endure these methods for a long period of time, get to the point where they rather die than having to support these therapies.

Juices made using a juice extractor are extremely healthy not only because they give you a nutritional boost of energy but also because you are able to ingest large amounts of fruits and vegetables in one serving and nourish every cell of your body with lots of vitamins, minerals and nutrients. When certain fruits and vegetables are combined in a single juice serving, they can increase the efficiency of the immune system, help with migraine headaches and detox your body. Most people don't like making juice using a juice extractor because they have to deal with all the cleaning involved with this type of machine. Another reason is that they've heard from other people that they don't really taste that good, or they just don't like the idea of drinking fruits and vegetables combined in a juice. Others believe that this type of juice therapy is too expensive. In reality if you replace all your meals with juicing for 10 days to get an overall body cleansing you will notice that juicing is actually cheaper than regular meals. This is the case if you take into account the electricity used to cook, the water you spend washing dishes, pots, spoons, etc., plus the time it takes to prepare the food and the food that gets spoiled each week (this happens in every home). However, if you are someone who eats canned food or microwave "meals" then you need more than just a cleansing because your body is probably malnourished and lacking the proper vitamins and minerals. By cleansing,

I'm talking about a "Liquid Cleanse". This is perhaps the most healthy and safe way of cleansing your body. This type of cleansing means juicing for breakfast, lunch and dinner for 10 consecutive days or at least 4 days if you don't think you can do it for 10 days. During this period you should not eat anything, even salads or fruits. This cleansing helps the liver and other organs recover and detoxify from the many years of eating the wrong foods. Believe me, this simple 10 day change can make wonders to all the cells in your body. As a matter of fact, I guarantee you that if you do this for ten consecutive days, you can lose between 15 to 20 pounds. If you continue juicing longer than this you will continue to lose weight until you hit your ideal weight. But in order to not fall off the wagon and get discourage about juicing, my recommendation is for you to do the ten day cleanse and then just replace one daily meal with juicing and eventually incorporate a whole day liquid diet once a week. However, juicing should be part of your daily routine or at least 3-4 times per week to keep your body properly nourished. Juicing can also help with migraine headaches, depression, and even lower blood pressure and glucose. Make sure you add a few green leafy vegetables like kale, wheat grass, celery, cucumber to balance the higher glycemic index of carrots, apples and other sweet fruits. If you want to see and feel the difference before and after this ten day cleanse, I recommend you to get a blood test before you start and after the ten days to feel the victory and achievement of your amazing effort.

Juice therapy is very healthy as it has been proven that this type of juice is absorbed quickly and easily, and best of all, they leave no residue in the intestine. These juices have exemplary nutritional qualities as the fruits and vegetables contain compounds that are vital to the human body. These juices help transporting proteins, minerals, enzymes, vitamins and water directly into the blood stream. Do your best to buy organic fruits and vegetables. It is true that these are more expensive than the conventional ones, but the nutritional value of organic products is higher than conventional. Also, the fact that they are not sprayed with herbicides, fungicides and other chemicals that are harmful to your health makes them a healthier choice and better for disease prevention. If you juice with non-organic fruits and vegetables, you may experience unfavorable health effects during the first 4 days. That could be a side effect of the chemicals they spray on these produce to keep them away from insects and other common pests. These chemicals also damage the ground because they lower the amount of potassium, magnesium, iron and calcium in the soil. So don't be surprised if you get a little sick when you are doing a liquid diet with these fruits and vegetables because these chemicals are extremely harmful. To make matters worse, in several countries including USA, Argentina, Colombia and others, some vegetables are genetically modified (GMO's) which can have dangerous health consequences such as cancer and arthritis. In the next chapter I explain in more detail these organisms and their possible side effects to your health. Many of the degenerative diseases are part of the worst statistics in the world, but especially in the United States where these have risen disproportionately since the introduction of genetically modified foods.

Now let's talk a little further about liquid cleansing and why it is very important for everyone. A juice-based cleansing will help to clean the liver, colon, skin and other body organs. If you suffer from weight gain or obesity, this cleanse will help you lose weight and depending on your focus and dedication, you may get to your ideal weight in a very short period of time. Please note that this doesn't happen overnight because if you have 40 extra pounds due to poor diet for several years, it wouldn't be fair to expect you to lose those 40 pounds in a week time frame, right? But I have heard of people losing up to 50 pounds in 2 months just by drinking juices from a juice extractor. This is what Joe Cross did in his documentary "Fat, Sick and Nearly Dead". I highly recommend this film if you're thinking about juicing to lose weight. By the way, adding exercise is vital to losing weight so make sure you add some type of exercise when you're doing this liquid diet.

The main purpose of liquid cleansing is to clear the mucus slush from the body to rid the body of toxins, bacteria and cysts accumulated for many years. Most diseases are curable but it depends on the person. There is no drug that cures any disease, that's a fact and it cannot be denied or challenged by the pharmaceutical industry. Drugs only take the pain away or treat a disease to make the person feel better but they don't provide a permanent cure. The only thing that can actually cure almost any disease is your own body. If the body is in complete balance, the immune system will work as it is designed to do, which is to eliminate any unwanted bacteria or viruses that try to enter or invade the body. It also works by supplying defenses will that help you fight diseases that invade the body through the skin, nose, mouth and other body parts. Another great benefit and perhaps the most important one to highlight from a liquid cleansing diet is that it raises the pH of the body and takes it to an alkaline level. Later I will explain the importance of an alkaline pH in the body and the foods that raise this vital marker of alkalinity. This balance can be obtained through good diet based on foods that are free of toxins, pesticides and carcinogens found in the many processed foods sold today. But the best way to bring your body to the proper balance is through juice therapy as these juices deliver nutrients, vitamins and minerals directly into the blood stream. These juices will help clear mucus from the body, which is related to the development of tumors, cysts and other toxins that accelerate the aging of tissues and cells. The mucus also promotes allergies, headaches and migraines.

One of the best ways to alkalize your juice is by adding organic celery to every juice you make. Celery is one of the most hydrating foods and because it is amazingly alkalizing, it balances you body's pH. Hundreds of years ago celery was used as an herb to treat many different health complaints. Celery is high in vitamin A and it is an excellent source of vitamins B1, B2, B6 and C. It has potassium, folic acid, calcium, magnesium, iron, sodium and essential amino acids. Celery is known to contain about 8 different anti-cancer compounds. A study from Rutgers University in New Jersey confirmed this by proving that celery prevents cancer cells from spreading. This characteristic may be attributed to a compound called acetylenics which stops the growth of tumor cells. There are a few other compounds in celery that prevent free radicals from damaging cells and prevent the formation of cancer cells. Celery also lowers cholesterol, aids digestion, lowers blood pressure, helps with weight loss, insomnia. It also helps eliminate and prevent urinary and gall bladder stones and the potassium and sodium help regulate kidney function and stimulate urine production.

Juice therapy also helps with a high consumption of fruits and vegetables that are essential to the health of internal and external organs. Many of the people who complete a liquid cleansing benefit from a bright and vivid skin because an internal cleansing is expressed in a positive way to the skin, eyes and hair.

Before starting the liquid cleansing I want you to know that during the cleanse you should not drink any milk or eat cheese, meat, chicken or any other meat. Nor should you eat processed foods and refined carbohydrates. You practically have to stop chewing for the duration of this liquid diet. The longer the duration of this diet is the longer the benefit and the faster the results that are achieved for any disease. As I said before, there are clinics in the USA, Mexico and other countries where juice therapy is used to treat serious diseases. The power of juice therapy is truly amazing and after many years of being in the dark side I am glad to see that people are finally realizing the miraculous benefits of juicing.

To start this cleansing, you have to be aware that it will not be easy and requires a lot of discipline; but I assure you that the benefit you will get from this is so incredible that you will feel renewed and satisfied to have achieved it. Your health depends on your dedication and commitment to give your body what it is asking for a long time, a cleanse. The first 3 or 4 days are perhaps the most difficult, but once you reach this initial milestone, your body will thank you when you begin to notice the loss of toxins and reduction or elimination of headaches and migraines. Gradually you will notice that the "appetite" or the feeling of stomach fatigue fades out and that has the always welcome effect of weight loss. You will also notice that the desperation and anxiety to cravings which most people are normally accustomed to decreases to the point that the body doesn't even miss it. This is important because certain cravings for sweets and highly processed treats are one of the causes of overweight, allergies and headaches.

Once you get past this 4 day grace period, you feel like you want to continue with this juicing therapy because people start to notice weight loss and most importantly, higher energy. To vary the routine of juicing, start adding some fiber to your diet by incorporating homemade smoothies (without cow's milk, please). In the appendix you will find some recipes for homemade juicing and smoothies to help you gain the benefits of a good liquid diet. These recipes will help you plan the consumption of juicing and smoothies for breakfast, lunch and dinner. These smoothies should be made with water or orange juice or grapefruit juice (preferably fresh squeezed at home) and not with cow's milk. In a later chapter I explain the dangers of cow's milk. These smoothies provide the benefit of fiber and protein along with the vitamins, minerals and nutrients that the fruits and vegetables provide. Some experts recommend drinking the smoothies in the morning and juicing for lunch and dinner. The best option is to avoid chewing anything during this period, but if you think this is an incentive to stay on this diet, I recommend eating healthy organic fruits, almonds, Brazil nuts, celery, carrots, green salads without creamy dressings and other vegetables.

Now, the question that you may be asking is for how many days do I have to do this liquid diet? To answer this question I first want to say that before you follow the recommendations of this book, you have to consult your family doctor to make sure you are a good candidate for this liquid diet. Unfortunately many doctors know very little about the benefits of juicing because the US medical education system doesn't require students to complete nutrition classes as part of the core curriculum. Most classes are related to the diagnosis of a disease and the medication to treat it. This is why many doctors are unaware of the healing powers of good nutrition in the form of juicing and smoothies. Once you feel confident and safe to do this diet and take advantage of its great benefits, you have to experiment with different fruits and vegetables to learn which combinations will best fit your organism. As I said before, every person is different and you have to listen to your body; if something doesn't sit well in your stomach, stop and try other combinations. No need to worry much about this because most people readily absorb and metabolize almost all combinations of these juices. There are many books and juicing guides that explain which combination of fruits and vegetables provide the best benefits for different goals. At the end of this book I suggest some options that can help you with this liquid diet. I recommend that you look for other combinations yourself to make this diet more enjoyable and to encourage you to continue and stay focused to the end. Educate yourself of the great benefits that this therapy provides you and remember that disease prevention based on good nutrition is a lot cheaper than treating chronic diseases caused by poor nutrition and lifestyle choices. It is my opinion and the opinion of many experts, scientists and doctors that juicing can save your life and may even cure chronic and terminal diseases such as cancer and heart disease. The key is to be consistent and change the bad foods that for many years have been accumulating small tumors or plaques in the arteries. Remember that 20 or 30 years of poor diet and lifestyle are not cured with 2 or 3 weeks of juicing. That will be very unrealistic. Those with advanced diseases, for example, need to make drastic changes to their diet and nutrition so their cells, organs, hormones and all metabolic functions are restored and back to performing their normal functions. The change in diet and the introduction of juice extracts can have a miraculous effect on your body that will amaze you and change your life forever. Finally and to re-iterate, I want to emphasize that organic produce are the most recommended for this liquid diet since they are not exposed to all kinds of chemicals such as fungicides, pesticides or herbicides. The seeds of these fruits and vegetables are not genetically modified in a laboratory as often happens with some of the conventional fruit and vegetables.

Enjoy your juice and smoothies and CHEERS!

GMO'S
GENETICALLY MODIFIED ORGANISMS

This is one of the hottest topics at this time because the FDA, for some reason, does not require food companies or multi-national chemical company giants like Monsanto, to label their products when they are made with genetically modified ingredients. If you do a quick internet search for the acronym GMO, you will realize that there are millions of articles and a number of scientific studies indicating that these are harmful to human health and should not be in the market as an alternative for organic or natural foods. According to several studies, these organisms have been linked with infertility problems, food allergies, resistance to antibiotics, gastrointestinal problems, liver damage and even cancer risks.

The European Union requires that all food manufactured with GMO's have their corresponding labels for the consumers to know what they are buying and decide for themselves whether to buy such foods or just say NO to GMO's. Moreover, in Asian countries like South Korea, Japan and even China it is also mandatory to label all packaged products containing GMO ingredients. In the United States, however, this requirement doesn't exist and consumers are virtually blind when buying food. According to FDA policy since 1992, foods with GMO's are no different than foods without it. It appears that the FDA doesn't listen or take into account the myriad of scientific studies that indicate the opposite. GMO's have been commercially available since 1994 and since then, the production of these foods has increased at an alarming rate. Over 90% of corn, cotton and soybeans produced in the United States are genetically modified. The now famous canola oil is also genetically modified. For this reason, when buying these products you should always buy organic or those with the "Non-GMO Project verified" logo. In case you didn't know, most processed foods are made from corn or soybeans; just read the back of the label and see for yourself. This means that almost all processed foods consumed in the USA contain close to 85% of these genetically lab made ingredients.

Unfortunately it is believed that this is the reason allergy rates have soared in the past 15 years. According to several experts on this subject, the percentage of certain food allergies increased to 18% in the period 1997 to 2007. As expected, one of the allergy research agencies said this was purely coincidental. Many of the studies done by independent groups say otherwise. This rate is now higher than 18%. If you are 40 years old or older, I'm sure you remember that allergies weren't as prominent 20-25 years ago. You hear of people with allergies almost every day today.

United States is the leader in these genetic plantations totaling approximately 70 million hectares in 2010. Every year companies like Monsanto are expanding their agenda to other countries to have full control of soybeans, corn and others. For those who don't know, Monsanto has patents on these seeds and no one can use them, Those who do either knowingly or by accident, are sued and prosecuted by law and forced to burn all their crops and pay fines and jail time. Please see the documentary "FOOD Inc.". This explains in more detail this issue of patented seeds. I don't know about you but I don't believe it should be legal for ANY company to have a patent to manufacture the basic raw material of most foods such as soy and corn. Food companies do their best to make the process as cheap as possible and to make sure the profits are as high as possible to keep their shareholders happy. When this happens, their mission or their incentive to produce healthy food is not their highest priority. For those who don't know, companies must reduce costs year after year because the cost of raw materials, overall production costs and employee salaries rise each year. This means that companies reduce food quality through new process technologies and many of these choose to change from natural and organic ingredients to synthetic and sometimes toxic chemicals that taste the same but could cause illness and allergies.

The damage it causes is yet to be seen, but what is well known is the health statistics of Americans, which is not very healthy at all. Some of these indicate that the rate of obesity, diabetes, Alhzeimer's, cancer and others has dramatically increased in the last decade or two. For example, one in four children has an increased level of obesity, one in two Americans die of cardiovascular disease and one in three dies of cancer. These are just a few. The saddest thing of all this is that the agencies that were created to regulate and take care of the health of Americans don't realize the issue at hand or simply don't want to hear any of these statistics nor the countless studies linking the diseases to certain foods and medicines. It is as if there was a plot or a partnership between these agencies (FDA, USDA) and the large food and drug companies. In my opinion, this is exactly the case.

The American Society of Nephrology, says the total number of deaths associated with acute renal (kidney) failure requiring dialysis rose from 18,000 in the year 2000 to 39,000 in the year 2009. This number is more than doubled in a decade. Several studies in laboratory animals show that in only 90 days, a diet with foods containing GMO's, the animals developed renal failure and other problems in their organs. Coincidence? I don't believe so. It doesn't take a genius to realize that there is a correlation between GMO's and organ damage. A study published by the International Journal of Biological Sciences which analyzes the effects of foods containing GMO's, found that Monsanto corn is linked to organ damage in laboratory rats; particularly damage to the kidneys, liver, and others.

I don't want to scare you with all this information but I do want to make you aware of these studies for you to make wise decisions based on studies published in scientific and medical journals. If for any reason you choose to ignore this information, I suggest that you at least do it for your children. The healthy future of these children or their future illnesses is in your hands; do not wait until the FDA or other government health institutions do their job the right way because you will be waiting a long time for that to happen.

To conclude this chapter, I want to summarize really quick and remind you that in more than 60 countries around the world there are significant restrictions or bans on genetically modified foods. Some of these countries are Japan, China, Russia, Mexico, Brazil, Bolivia, Peru and most of the countries in the European Union. However, in the United States and Canada, there are no restrictions on these foods or mandates on labeling these foods. Furthermore, in the 2012 elections here in the United States, companies like Monsanto, Coca-Cola, Dow Corning and a few others, invested more than US$45 million in campaigning to make sure Proposition # 37 didn't pass in California. The purpose of this proposal was to force food companies and chemical companies to put labels on any product containing GMO ingredients so that consumers could have the option to buy or reject those foods.

Unfortunately those $45 million dollars were able to convince most people to vote against such labels. I find it completely absurd that in such a powerful country like the United States, the land of the free, we have to vote for something as fundamental as labeling the foods we eat so we can make a smart buying decision. Why do we have to beg these companies to let us know what's in their foods? I don't want my family to be part of this grand experiment that the food and drug companies are doing, I should have the right to know which foods contain GMO's. If the rest of the population wants to eat those foods, that's their choice and I'm totally okay with that. Unfortunately, the FDA and the government seem to care very little about people getting sick or dying because of GMO's. It seems like the law makers in Congress are more interested in the well being of these companies than you and I, perhaps because eventually these companies will contribute large amounts of money for their political campaigns. In many cases, these companies have hired the same politicians who were supposed to be regulating their foods or drugs, for top pay jobs. These companies like to hire these politicians and FDA top officials because they will eventually help them get their foods and drugs approved quicker since they have very good connections in these government agencies. Sad, very sad indeed.

FDA APPROVED DRUGS

On this subject I can probably write an entire book of 300 pages, but in this book I will explain the most important and the most dangerous drugs. This is a topic that no one wants to talk about. No one dares to get into the details of the dangers and side effects they have on people, especially those who take them for several months or years. For some reason, the Media, Politicians, the FDA and in some cases, doctors don't want to talk about this subject. As I said before, according to statistics from the Center for Disease Control, medicines approved by the FDA and properly prescribed by medical doctors, end the lives of approximately 100,000 people each year, in the United States alone. This number is equivalent to almost two football stadiums completely filled with people and suddenly vanishing. Amazing right? Do you remember when the 911 terrorists attacked the twin towers in New York in 2001? Who can forget that day? Well, that day, just over 3,000 innocent people died and the United States declared war to global terrorism. We all know the rest of the history which we still live to this day. However, why doesn't the government arrest anyone from the pharmaceutical companies that sell deadly drugs? Why doesn't the government punish the FDA for approving these drugs which are killing thousands of people each year? If these drugs are killing more than 100,000 Americans each year because of their side effects, why doesn't the FDA raise a BIG red flag and say something about it? I don't know about you but 100,000 people per year is a tragedy of GREAT magnitudes. Did you know that prescription drugs have a higher percentage of deadly car crashes than alcohol and marihuana? Why doesn't anybody dare to talk about this? Only a group of independent entities like Naturalnews.com, Food Democracy Now and the book "The 24 hour Pharmacist" by Suzy Cohen, dare to talk about it in radio and television interviews. It's sad that this is happening every year but the media doesn't seem to care. I wonder why the national network channels do not cover this news as the biggest News Alert of the century or talk about it every day for a week or two so people see and hear that this is a tragedy that needs to be addressed. Why do they make such a big fuss about the flu vaccine each year or the swine flu virus back then? They make sure everyone knows that the flu vaccine is available and everyone should get it and if they don't, the consequences could be fatal; which is not true. But they don't tell the public that the side effects of these vaccines can actually be fatal, because in many cases the vaccines are more dangerous than beneficial. There is no evidence that vaccines are effective. The literature that comes with these vaccines makes it clear that there is no correlation between the presence of an anti-virus and protection against a disease. So it seems like someone assumed that if a substance is applied to the body and the body develops an antibody to this substance, then the person is immune and will not get sick. This is completely false because the immune system is very complex and it can be compromised if there are several factors present at the time of an external attack like a contaminant. For example, if a person gets the flu vaccine and that person eats poorly or is more exposed to contact with other people who have the flu, or has a very high stress level, that person will get sick even if he or she was given 2 or 3 flu vaccines. Now, if a person eats healthy, has no stress and has little contact with sick people, chances are that person will never get sick. I give this example because I have never gotten the flu shot and I can say that in the past 8 years that I've been eating healthy, I have not been infected with the so called "Flu", even though I work in a building with more than 300 people with central air conditioning re-circulating the sneezes and coughs of all those who already carry the flu and other contagious illnesses. This means that the problem is not in the virus or the disease, the problem lies in the health of the individual and how compromised is the medium in which he lives.

There are an infinite number of medicines that have been recalled because they have caused thousands of deaths and the FDA was left with no choice but to force the pharmaceutical companies to stop selling such medicines. In this part of the book I provide you with just a few of them but believe me, the number of these medicines is much higher and I urge you to educate yourself on a particular drug that you or a love one may be taking so you understand its side effects and talk to your doctor to help compensate for the side effects or ask the doctor to change it. Become a smart patient and don't let your doctor be the only decision maker when it comes to your health because at the end of the day, it is your body and no one knows your body more than yourself.

VIOXX

Let's start with Vioxx. This drug was one of the most sold medicines in the United States with sales approaching $ 2.6 billion dollars a year. This drug was prescribed to people with chronic and acute body aches and pains associated with arthritis. After a mountain of evidence that clearly indicated that this drug was causing thousands of deaths from heart attacks and strokes, the maker of this drug, MERCK, recalled it after five years of its approval by the Food and Drug Administration. However, this drug had already killed an estimated number of 60,000 people and caused permanent damage to about 140 thousand people according to an article by the respected and well known Doctor Mercola in May 2012. The highlight of this is that it wasn't the FDA that forced the company to withdraw this drug from the market. It was MERCK itself that recalled it after the amount of evidence presented by doctors, hospitals and independent groups. This forced Merck to initiate an internal clinical study that showed clearly that the side effects of this drug were extremely dangerous and fatal. My question is, why didn't the FDA do it when the evidence was presented to them by independent health advocacy groups? Makes you think doesn't it?

At a congressional hearing in 2005, evidence showed that Merck knew of the fatal effects of Vioxx related to heart attacks. During this hearing Merck was asked why they didn't instruct their sales people to mention the side effects on heart attacks. This company actually ensured them that this drug had minimal risks. This may be proof that the current marketing of medicines is full of deceit and lies to sell their drugs quickly, regardless of the damage they cause to society.

"The more than 3,000 sales representatives of the company MERCK are trained in an extraordinary way to capitalize any interaction with the doctors," said California Representative Henry Waxman, during the congressional hearing. "But when it came to the information that the doctors needed the most about VIOXX according to their risk - MERCK responses appear to be disinformation and censorship," Representative

Waxman said.

Dr. David Graham who was a safety researcher at the FDA high command center said the following at a US congressional hearing "The FDA does not have the ability to protect Americans." The FDA just doesn't have the ability to fully study all the medicines and foods that need to be approved by this agency. One thing that most people don't know is that the FDA has no laboratories to test ANY of the foods and drugs they approve year after year. They base their approvals on studies supplied by the pharmaceutical and food companies. This is like taking a math test with all the answers next to you and getting a 100% in your final score. In my opinion, none of this agency's approvals are effective or safe and they actually put your life in danger.

AVANDIA

Let's continue with the drug linked to more than 10,000 deaths related to heart attacks, strokes and permanent liver damage. Since the drug was approved in 1999, GSK said it was effective and safe if properly used. However, a plethora of independent studies showed that this drug was extremely dangerous and its risks did not justify the low benefits. Studies conducted by GSK in 2011-2012 showed that evidently this drug increased the risk of heart attacks and strokes. But GSK already knew this since 1999, because their own documents that surfaced during an investigation confirmed what many independent studies claimed. But instead of publishing the results and alert the FDA, this company spent 11 years trying to cover this evidence. In addition, the United States Senate accused GSK of not publishing another study by the same company in 2003 which clearly showed that more heart patients died when they took this drug than those who took a placebo pill. A placebo is a sugar pill, a fake treatment or a shot that misleads patients into thinking they are taking a real medicine when in fact they are taking a fake pill. This is done for scientific comparison and trials of a certain drug.

Glaxo-Smith-Kline had impressive sales of nearly $ 3.2 billion dollars in 2006 alone. According to an FDA scientist an approximate number of 100,000 heart attacks were attributed to this drug and increased the risk of heart attacks by 43%. The FDA knew about these risks since 2007 but despite the evidence and instead of removing it from the market, the FDA let the drug continue selling with the condition that the side effect insert that comes with the drug had a small note indicating the danger of this drug. As expected, thousands of people died between 2007 and 2012 when the drug was finally withdrawn from the market. I ask this question over and over again.....Why did the FDA take so long to recall such a dangerous drug even when they had so much evidence of its risks? The sad part of this is that no one went to jail because the company GlaxoSmithKline and other drug companies are not a "Person" but instead they are corporations that are protected by many loop holes in the federal laws. All the deaths go unpunished. The only thing that happens is a lawsuit that normally takes years to process and since it is very difficult to prove that a certain medication caused permanent damage or death, some of these lawsuits get dismissed. Some others, however, get processed but the amount of money these companies have to pay is minimal compared to the billions of dollars they make in profit during the time the drug is under its patent. Speaking of which, this drug's patent expired in 2012. Is this why the FDA didn't take action in previous years? Did the lobbyists of this company convince the FDA to allow them to continue selling this drug until the patent expired? It makes you think, doesn't it? Maybe it's hard to believe, but it seems that the FDA doesn't act on behalf of the patients but instead of the interest of these pharmaceuticals that in my opinion only care about their shareholders instead of the health of the patients. What's worse is that the FDA doesn't respond to any government laws and they are free of any regulatory scrutiny. They actually elect their own leaders and executives. This is probably why most of these agents are now working as senior managers and executives for large pharmaceutical, food and chemical corporations. It also happens the other way around. Don't you think these executives would be involved in some kind of conflict of self-interest when they have to approve a drug or food from these giant corporations? In my opinion, this is exactly what happens and that's why I don't trust the transparency of the FDA, CDC, USDA and others. There seems to be some kind of favoritism to certain corporations because they know that eventually one of these companies is going to offer them a high rank position with a very attractive salary.

MIRENA IUD

This is an intrauterine contraceptive in the form of a "T" of small size that is inserted into the uterus by a licensed doctor. This contraceptive is implanted for a period of up to 5 years to prevent pregnancy.

Many side effects have been reported since the introduction of this device to the market. Some of these are minor such as infection or inflammation of the pelvis. Some complications are more severe and can lead to serious problems. These include perforation of the uterus, cervix and intestines. In some cases this device has to be removed by surgery because it can move to other internal body parts. The following are some of the side effects of this drug according to its own documentation: bleeding or abnormal bleeding not related to the period, increased blood sugar, ovarian cysts, enlargement of an ovary, low energy, dizziness, water retention, severe stomach pains, diarrhea, vomiting, depression, breast pain, hair loss, low sex drive or desire for sex, insomnia and acne.

Remember that this contraceptive like every single medicine prescribed by a doctor or sold at a pharmacy has to be approved by the FDA and therefore most people trust that they are perfectly safe. Unfortunately that is not the case and as I explained before, many people die or suffer permanent damage because of some of the side effects of these FDA approved drugs.

Something that I find utterly inexplicable is the fact that most people are concerned about purchasing life insurance, car insurance and health insurance as prevention tools. Most people apply sun screen to protect themselves from sunlight and they even buy health insurance for a pet. However, these same people don't care about healthy eating to give their body a natural and free health insurance. I often tell my friends and family not to drink sodas (regular or diet), or avoid drinking homogenized and pasteurized milk; and the answer I often get is something like "we have to die of something" That's true, but what they don't take into account is the fact that the last years of their life can be miserable not only for themselves but for their loved ones who have to take care them until the their last breath. Think about it, nobody wants to be a burden to their loved ones. They have their own problems and their families to deal with. With our aim to achieve a healthy life style, isn't it better to get older and be able to deal with life without having to depend on someone else?
You and I know that one, two or three sodas won't kill you, but the slow damage being done is monumental and permanent. The worst part is that the older a person is (after 50) the fewer the cells his or her body produces and the faster the physical decline. Remember my advice…...Prevention is a thousand times better than medication.

ZOLOFT

Before you start taking this medication, I want to ask you one thing.....Don't you think it is very normal to sometimes feel sad, lonely, angry or anxious for any number of reasons? Well I'm sorry to tell that the health system in the United States believes that these emotions are not normal and you have to be medicated with very dangerous Psychotic drugs which can be highly detrimental to your mental and physical health.

Zoloft is one of the most commonly prescribed medicines for depression in the world. This is part of the family of medicines called Selective Serotonin Reuptake Inhibitors or SSRI's. Other drugs in this family are Prozac, Luvox, Lexapro, Paxil and others. These medicines have very dangerous side effects.

Sales of this type of medication were nearly $ 10 billion dollars in 2010 in the USA alone. These drugs are prescribed "normally" to people over 60 years of age. Note how I put quotes between the word "normally" to emphasize that in my opinion it should not be normal to prescribe these medicines to anyone. One reason is that this medication is prescribed to this demographic group of people is because they visit their doctors when they feel depressed, lonely and sad after their spouse dies or when they are alone for a long time and have no family members to share the last years of their lives. Here in the United States is very common to see elderly people in nursing homes completely abandoned by their loved ones. It is unfortunate to see these elderly people live alone without frequent visits from their children, grandchildren and other relatives. The Hispanic, Italian and Asian cultures are very different in this regard as most prefer to have their parents or grandparents at home until their last breath. Obviously there are exceptions in all these cultures.

In many cases, these drugs should not be prescribed because this type of depression is normal. The best remedy for these people is to find them something to do such as hobbies and other alternatives to make them laugh, exercise, stay active and be part of the community to fill those gaps that will help them feel alive and part of society. The solution in these cases is not to medicate them with dangerous depression drugs. I want you to know one of the main side effects of these drugs, suicidal and homicidal thoughts; these are very common in most people taking these medications. Moreover, many of the heinous acts of violence that have occurred in recent years in the United States and the world, have been perpetrated by people taking this type of medication. So don't you think that if one of the side effects of these drugs is suicidal thoughts, it is very dangerous to prescribe these medications? And that it is very likely that the medicines could be the cause of the alarming number of suicides and homicides which the media doesn't care to cover? Therefore, no one is aware of these highly harmful side effects and society doesn't see the connection between these violent acts and this type of drugs. According to the recent statistics involving American soldiers from the Afghanistan and Iraq wars, more soldiers die by suicide here in the United States than those who die fighting. But no one questions the medical system in this country. No one brings the debate of the possible connection between these drugs and the number of suicides from soldiers diagnosed with post war depression syndrome and other post war dramatic situations. In 2012 for example, 303 soldiers committed suicide and 212 were killed in combat in Afghanistan. The latest statistics indicate that an average of 22 soldiers commit suicide daily in the United States.

Another very serious issue is the fact that many people don't even know that these medications have never been tested in children under 18 years of age so these children are basically the guinea pigs for this type of drugs. Nonetheless, it is very common in the US to prescribe such drugs to children who have been diagnosed with Attention Deficit Hyperactivity Disorder or ADHD. In my opinion and that of several scientists and experts in the field, this "disease" was invented as part of a huge pharmaceutical marketing campaign to sell these drugs to a younger demographic. Remember that these medicines were originally created for people over 60 years of age. Dr. Peter Breggin, MD, who wrote the book called Toxic Psychiatry, describes a very disturbing study published in the American Journal of Psychiatry in February 1990, where six depressed patients who were free of any suicidal thoughts before taking Prozac, developed violent thoughts and suicide attempts after taking this drug for only two to seven weeks. Some of these thoughts lasted from three days to three months after they stop taking this medicine. In August 1990, Dista Products Company which is a division of Eli Lilly added suicidal thoughts in a pamphlet for doctors explaining the danger of this medicine and its connection to this dangerous side effect. The big question is ….. Why doesn't the FDA take action on the matter and investigate these medicines a little more in depth? Don't put too much thought to this question because in my opinion the answer is …..The FDA will not withdraw any of these drugs from the market until the patent expires. This is because pharmaceutical companies will lose a lot of money if that were to happen. Also remember that the FDA is the agency that approves all drugs sold in the USA and pulling too many drugs from the market will damage its reputation and its efficacy will be questioned. So just remember that the prescribed and over the counter medicines that you take or give to your children may not be tested or proven to be safe by the FDA other than just reviewing the pharmaceutical's own studies. In addition, the FDA requires these companies to only submit two positive studies even if the company has to perform several studies (5 to 10) to be able to get 2 positive ones. In other words, if 8 of the 10 studies are negative, the FDA only cares about the 2 positive studies these companies submit to them. This agency is proud to say that the United States has the most advanced pharmaceutical system in the world. If this is true, why do over one hundred thousand people die every year from taking FDA approved drugs? Why does the United States spend more money than any other country in the world in health care (which I call, sick care) but ranks last in longevity among 16 other industrialized countries including Japan, Australia, Switzerland and Norway? Think about it, the United States has more obese and sick people than any other country in the world. It is very likely that food and drugs are the main cause of this tragedy. Nobody looks at the root cause of the problem even though 80% of the "foods" sold in the United States are processed. There is something fundamentally wrong in the health care of America where big food and big pharma are making Billions of dollars from the fat and sick people of this wonderful country. How much longer do we have to wait for politicians to realize that their approvals and decisions in Congress are making people fatter and sicker year after year?

STATIN DRUGS (Cholesterol drugs)

Statins drugs are those approved to lower total cholesterol. These are in my opinion one of the worst prescription drugs in the world. For some reason, cholesterol was named the bad guy a while ago. Today everyone talks about cholesterol like a cancer that must be eradicated immediately. Little do they know that cholesterol is extremely essential to health; that is why the body manufactures it in the liver. A very low cholesterol is more dangerous than high cholesterol. According to studies on this subject, low cholesterol is responsible for thousands of deaths annually in the United States. A Japanese study found that men with cholesterol levels below 161 mg / dl had an increased mortality rate of 49% associated with stroke, heart failure and cancer. Women had a 50% increase in mortality for the same reason. However, those with cholesterol levels near 242 mg / dl did not have any risk of death. This kind of study is constantly ridiculed by the medical system and every time a doctor or scientist comes out and contradicts any study created for the benefit of a certain medicine, this doctor is threatened with losing his/her license or is ridiculed by the system with the help of the national news media by questioning their credibility in the scientific community.

Why were Statin drugs created? Some time ago several scientists and doctors met and concluded that a cholesterol reading over 200 mg/dl was dangerous because it could lead to plaque in the artery walls. According to many scientific studies and independent groups this is simply not true. What is true is that a diet high in saturated animal fat such as milk, meat, poultry and others, is associated with increased levels of bad cholesterol or LDL, which helps to create plaque in the arteries and eventually raise blood pressure. Scientists and doctors who support and confirm that a total cholesterol above 200 mg/dl is very dangerous to human health and can cause heart disease, do not understand why there are thousands of people in the world that have cholesterol levels higher than 400 mg/dl and in certain people up to 600 mg/dl without heart problems or other heart disease related issues. Rodrigo, my brother's brother-in-law, for example, had a total cholesterol over 2000 mg/dL and his triglycerides level was over 1500 mg/dL over 10 years ago. His levels were so high that the doctor could not believe he was still alive with such readings. He was asked to repeat the blood tests to be sure that there was no error. Realizing that it wasn't a mistake, he was sent to a special treatment in the laboratories of a prestigious University in Miami, Florida. He was prescribed Statin drugs to lower cholesterol and triglycerides but after taking these drugs for a while, Rodrigo realized that the effects of this medication kept him weak and his muscles were sore more often than before taking this medication, which is one of the most common side effects of Statin drugs. He then started reading and educating himself about his case and realized that diet was a major cause of his condition. However, what helped him the most to lower his cholesterol and triglyceride levels besides changing some foods in his diet, was drinking lots of water. That's right, sounds simple but that's basically what changed his numbers. Now, I'm not talking about 6 to 8 cups of water; I'm talking about close to a gallon of water every day. Rodrigo hasn't taken any medicine to lower or control his cholesterol levels since about three years ago. His lipid profile numbers are now virtually controlled or in the normal range.

Like Rodrigo there are thousands of people around the world and especially in northern Italy where there is a village called Stocarreddo, near Venice, where 38% of the residents have total cholesterol levels above 600 mg/dL and yet they are not dropping dead or suffer from heart disease. Many people don't know, but cholesterol levels in dogs are higher than 400 mg/dL; however, they are not dying of heart attacks or at least not as often as humans. Cholesterol is actually very important to human health. Unless you have plaque buildup in your arteries, high cholesterol levels alone is not the main culprit in heart attacks. Low cholesterol levels are actually more dangerous to your health. Low cholesterol levels will cause your testosterone to drop and guess what will happen….you will need another drug to increase your testosterone levels. I wonder if that's the reason many men today are going to the doctor to get a prescription for low-T. I also wonder if the over prescription of cholesterol lowering medications in the past 20 years are actually causing this drastic low-T epidemic. A better and more efficient way to check if you are at risk of a heart attack is a test called "Homocysteine". This test should be a routine test prescribed alone with the normal lipid profile test. If this test is too high and your cholesterol levels are also high, then you may be at a higher risk of a heart attack.

Statin drugs have very dangerous side effects and you need to know them before you commit to taking this type of medications for a long period of time. Many independent scientists, clinics and some Doctors warn that these drugs can cause serious heart problems. This is ironic because one of the reasons people take these medications is to prevent heart disease. The main reason some Doctors warn about these drugs is because one of their side effects is to rob the co-enzyme CoQ10 from the liver to be able to work properly. This co-enzyme is responsible for keeping the heart active and with the energy it needs to keep pumping blood in a healthy way. 50mg of CoQ10 twice a day also decreases high blood pressure (Systolic) by 11% and low blood pressure (Diastolic) by 12%. When the level of CoQ10 decreases, the heart and all the muscles weaken. That's why people who are taking these medications feel very tired and have a lot of muscle pain or myalgia. Please note that the heart is also a muscle. Many European countries require that the small insert that comes nicely folded with these medications have a warning or precaution on the bottom called the little black box. This precaution is actually for doctors to inform their patients that they should take a certain amount of CoQ10 while taking Statins drugs. This helps replenish the levels of Co-Q10 that Statin drugs normally reduce. In the United States, however, the FDA does not require this kind of precaution despite the amount of data demonstrating the danger of not doing so. Other side effects of Statin drugs are type II diabetes, liver damage, erectile dysfunction, joint pain, diarrhea, stomach pain, liver toxicity, mood swings, difficulty sleeping or depression. There are other reported cases such as Rhabdomyolysis which involves the breakdown of muscle fibers. These fibers can be absorbed by the circulatory system and cause toxicity to the kidneys and can lead to kidney damage. Such is the case of the drug Cerivastatin which was withdrawn from the market for causing this muscle damage. Don't forget that this was another one of those FDA approved drugs. This is another reason I don't have high confidence on anything the FDA approves.

Another side effect is the possible damage that it causes to the liver since these medicines like most others depend on the liver to work effectively. As I mentioned before, medicines steal enzymes from the liver to do their job. If a patient doesn't eat well or doesn't replenish these enzymes and minerals, the liver begins to be deficient of these nutrients and requires the kidneys to work extra to help the liver. The problem gets worse if we add a high consumption of alcohol. This gradually causes the liver and the kidneys to become weaker and weaker until they fail and start to cause serious complications that eventually leads to permanent organ damage and death.

Another serious side effect of Statin drugs is Lou Gehrig's disease or Amyotrophic Lateral Sclerosis (or ALS). Remember the ice bucket challenge? The Wall Street Journal reported in July 2007 the possible connection of Statins and this disease. Okay, don't be alarmed and start panicking about the Statin drugs you may be taking at this time. Remember that every human body is different and these side effects don't affect 100% of the patients. Just monitor your body and let your doctor know of any symptoms you may experience while taking these drugs. The human body is a very complicated machine and has millions of chemical and biological reactions that work well or not so well depending on the food you eat, the environment you live in and your life style.

There are many supplements that are believed to lower cholesterol and help balance the lipid profile in a natural way without dangerous side effects. Among these supplements are Red yeast rice, Omega 3, Guggul (Indian plant), Ferulic Acid, Lecithin, Pumpkin Seed Oil, Quercetin A and ginger root. It is believed that the Indian plant Guggul also helps patients with arthritis, acne, hemorrhoids, urinary tract infections and even to encourage weight loss. A study of human cells in 2007 found that Guggul induced cell death of prostate cancer and a study in 2008 reported that Guggul reduced skin tumors in rats.

Before closing this topic, I want to add the following if you decide to stop taking your Statin medication. Please consult your family doctor before making this decision so he can determine whether you are a good candidate to stop this medication or continue taking it and just supplement it with CoQ10. I'm only providing you with the side effects that nobody reads and providing you with different alternatives for you to investigate further and take control of your health. Either way only you have the final decision to stop taking your medications and start taking supplements. Educate yourself by asking your doctor, reading scientific journal and most importantly reading the pamphlet that comes with your medication and those that your children may be taking. If you believe that doctors know everything and everything they recommend is the best for you or your children, I regret to inform you that they are human and as such they also make mistakes. They don't have time to keep current with all the different scientific findings and alternative treatments to most diseases and to top it off, the continuing education that most doctors receive is provided by the pharmaceutical companies which is no more than a great marketing campaign and a sales pitch to introduce a new drug to market. For this sales pitch, doctors are usually invited to very nice resorts with all expenses paid by the drug company. Please note that most doctors are very smart people and most of them studied medicine because they want to help their patients and make them feel better but unfortunately today's medical system is practically governed by the pharmaceutical industry and their potentially dangerous FDA approved drugs.

MY WISH AND MY CHALLENGE

In the next few pages I give you summarized information about different topics to make it easier for the reader to use as future reference and to better grasp the concepts. It contains statistical points and facts that will make you think. This information is concise and presented in bullet form to help you understand it better and apply it to your daily life. It is full of recommendations that may help you prevent and potentially cure many of the chronic and degenerative diseases that affect a great number of Americans today.

My wish is that you apply these recommendations and communicate them to your loved ones and friends so they can also enjoy a life full of physical, emotional and mental health. I hope you can help me convey this message of health and vitality to as many people as you can so together we can gradually reduce the death statistics in the United States and the world through prevention and good nutrition. It is my hope that one day drugs are only used in emergency cases or extreme situations. It is also my hope that medicines are not the first step to take when your child has a fever or a slight cough. I also hope that governments don't force or mandate vaccines. Vaccines should be voluntary and the government and medical authorities should educate their citizens by teaching them and highlighting the side effects and contraindications of vaccines and other drugs. I also hope that one day vaccines and drugs are made with ingredients that don't cause other diseases or even death as it is the case of some of them today. More on this subject in the vaccines chapter.

My challenge is trying to make people understand that drugs are not the solution for reaching optimum health and definitely not to cure a disease because they don't. I know it's difficult for people to get out of the "normal" health paradigm. That's what has been indoctrinated in all of us for the past 100 years and most people believe that there is no better way to prevent or cure diseases. Well, let me tell you that if you follow the herd you will be slaughtered. Don't believe everything you are told and if you choose not to believe the facts and points that I present in this book, that's okay; I actually want you to become an educated reader and consumer.

Read other books related to health and question everything including your most trusted doctor. Remember that ALL drugs or medicines have side effects and you need to know them before you start taking them so you understand and identify the side effects when you start to experience them. Most drugs, when taken long term, will create a vicious cycle of other drugs because the first drug you take will most likely cause another disease for which you will need another drug and so on and so forth.

If you believe FDA drugs are good, I challenge you or anyone who is taking 5-10 medications at this time to compare blood test results and your physical and state of mind with my test results (I don't take any medicines at all). If you are one of those people that believes medicine will help you stay 100% healthy and disease free; I am sorry to tell you that will never be the case. I know there is no person out there who is taking 5-10 medications and is 100% healthy; it's just not possible. I recommend you to be healthy through prevention by eating the proper foods that will nourish your body and help elevate your immune system. Medication will eventually cause lamentation later in life. Join me to discover the reason why people get sick, I invite you to enjoy this part of the book in a slideshow form to help you live life without pain and dangerous medicines. Following this program may help you stay free of diseases and be healthy for life. It will help you avoid being part of the negative statistics and potential side effects of the FDA approved medicines. Join me to live a healthy life until the last breath of your life.

As I mentioned before, talk to your doctor before making any changes to your diet or life style.

TOPICS TO COVER IN PRESENTATION FORM

- Ingredients in processed foods

- List of good and bad foods

- Importance of supplements

- Diseases and possible cures

- The importance of pH in the blood

    - Acidic food chart
    - Alkaline food chart

- Glycemic Index

    - Food chart with High, Medium and Low Glycemic Index

- Vaccines and their dangers

- Natural herbs and their healing powers

INGREDIENTS

- Hydrogenated Oils (Trans Fats)

- Omega 6 fats

- Monosodium Glutamate (MSG)

- High Fructose Corn Syrup or HFCS

- Artificial Colors, Flavors and Sweeteners

- Nitrates and Nitrites in processed meats

- Aluminum and Parabens in deodorants

Hydrogenated Oils or Trans Fats

These are extremely dangerous to your health and should be avoided at all cost. They have absolutely no benefit to humans or animals for that matter. They are produced in a lab introducing hydrogen to the fat when heated at very high temperatures. These fats are only beneficial to food companies because they are cheaper than natural fats and last much longer on store shelves. These fats are found in butter, cookies, ice cream, cream cheese, hundreds of processed foods and other products. Just read the labels.

- Increases LDL cholesterol which is the bad cholesterol

- Decreases HDL which is the good cholesterol

- Clog arteries that feed the brain and the heart

- It is the # 1 cause of heart disease

- Increases the risk of type II diabetes

- Increases the life of processed foods. This is only good for the companies not you

- Studies indicate that it causes cancer, heart attacks, diabetes, liver disease and obesity

- An increase of only 2% increases the risk of diabetes by 39%.

- It is basically a poison that causes the slow disintegration of all the cells in the body and gradually reduces mitochondria in cells.

- Causes high blood pressure, acne and infertility

- Helps create free radicals and promotes internal inflammation

- Reduces metabolism, perhaps because the cells harden

Statistics and facts

- One in two Americans die from heart disease each year

- Every 34 seconds a person dies from heart disease, this equates to about 2,500 people each day. Do you want to be part of these statistics?

- Every 20 seconds there is a heart attack

- Men suffer from a heart attack 10 years earlier than women

- A Harvard expert said: "If Trans fats are replaced with natural oils, that alone can prevent 30,000 deaths a year." I bet you didn't hear that on the news.

- Just one serving of small French fries contain the dietary value of 1.5 days worth of trans fats under the US nutritional diet rules

- According to Scientists and Naturopathic doctors the only safe portion of Trans Fats is ZERO

Omega 6

These fats are called essential fats and your body needs them to build healthy cells and maintain nerve and brain function. However, the typical American diet contains too much Omega 6 fats and hence should be reduced to reach an optimum balance. Omega 6 fats are everywhere in the food chain from crackers to GMO corn and soy. We consume too much Omega 6 because most of the processed foods contain some type of soy or corn base oils. The ideal ratio of omega 3 and omega 6 should be 1:1 but the standard American diet has a ratio of 1:20 omega 3 to omega 6 respectively. This is bad news because too much omega 6 and too little omega 3 can create havoc in your cells and tissues and cause internal inflammation which over stimulate your immune system. That's why there should always be a balance of these essential fats.

- Omega 6 fats are believed to be one of the main causes of breast cancer.

- Also called Polyunsaturated Fats.

- Studies indicate that they also cause obesity.

- High consumption increases the likelihood of almost all types of cancer by producing toxic compounds that feed cancer cells.

- These oils are also associated with heart attacks, arthritis, inflammation, depression and osteoporosis.

Sources:

Vegetable oils like safflower, corn, palm, sunflower, cottonseed and soybean oil. All of these can be found in most cookies, crackers, cakes, pastries, bagels, bread, muffins, doughnuts, pancakes, and many others. You need to read the ingredients on the back of the packages.

Monosodium Glutamate or MSG

- This is a Neurotoxin or Excitotoxin which causes cell death

- Attacks the brain barrier or membrane

- It sticks to tissues and creates free radicals

- Connected to diseases such as Alzheimer's and Parkinson's

- It was never tested in a laboratory but it was approved by the FDA in the same way that salt and pepper was approved

- FDA warns that MSG is harmful to children and the elderly. If this is the case, why doesn't the FDA just ban this ingredient?

- Dr. Schwartz says that two tablespoons of MSG on a piece of bread can kill a medium size dog in a matter of minutes

- In the 50's in the US, consumption was 12 gm/year per person. Today that number is 450 gm/year per person. Wow, and we wonder why Alzheimer's disease wasn't common in the 80's but today it is the #6 cause of death in the US. Coincidence? I don't believe so.

- Humans are 5 times more sensitive than rats. Studies have found that lab rats are negatively impacted by MSG and foods containing MSG

- MSG is hidden under more than 35 names. I list most of them in the next pages.

Ingredients that contain MSG

- Autolized Yeast
- Calcium Caseinate
- Gelatin
- Glutamate
- Glutamic Acid
- Soy Protein
- Soy Protein Isolate
- Hydrolized Protein
- Soy Protein Hydrolized
- Monopotasium Glutamate
- Sodium Caseinate
- Yeast Extract
- Yeast Nutrient
- Textured Protein
- Soy Sauce
- Soy Sauce Extract
- Pectin
- Plant Protein Extract
- Fortified Protein
- Condiments
- Seasonings

- Maltodextrin
- Carrageenan
- Corn Protein
- Whey Protein Isolate
- Whey Protein Concentrate
- Magnesium Glutamate
- Natural Flavors
- Malt Extract
- Malted Barley
- Soup helpers (cubes)
- Oligodextrin
- Bouillon Stock
- Broth Stock
- Natrium Glutamate
- Calcium Glutamate

- Corn Starch

Foods that contain MSG

- Jams

- Ham

- Bacon

- Pepperoni

- Bottled Juices

- Canned food

- Tofu (non-organic)

- Ice Cream

- Cake Mixes

- Cookies

- Bubble Gum

- Baby Formulas

- Dressings

- Sodas

- Cheese

People that are extra sensitive to MSG may react to these ingredients

- Yeast

- Brown rice syrup

- Citric acid

- Cornstarch

- Corn Syrup

- Butter Fat

- Lipolyzed butter fat

- Powdered milk

- Modified starch and modified food starch

- Nutritional Yeast

- Fortified Protein

- Enriched vitamins

- Reduced fat milk

Symptoms and diseases caused by MSG

- Addiction

- Allergies

- Alzheimer's

- Asthma Attacks

- Nerve Attacks

- Chest pain

- Depression

- Migraines

- Angina or Accelerated Palpitations

- Food cravings

- Confusion

- Neurological Disorders

- Breaking of Skin

- Stroke

- Shortness of breath

- Obesity and seizures

Statistics and facts

- Alzheimer's wasn't too common in the 80's, today is the #6 cause of death in the US with about 74,600 deaths annually

- 5.3 million people have Alzheimer's

- Asthma was uncommon in the 80's, today it kills 5,000 Americans annually and 180,000 worldwide.

- The number of prescriptions for ADHD has risen 500% since 1991.

- The number of suicides in China is 250,000 a year, or 42% of the world's suicide rate. China uses a lot of MSG in their food

- Type II Diabetes and obesity increased 10 times in five years in the US. MSG may be the cause due to cravings of the wrong foods

- American children are three times more likely to be prescribed psychotropic drugs than European children

High Fructose Corn syrup (HFCS)

- It contains lots of calories and can cause obesity

- Alters metabolism and increases the risk of developing type II diabetes

- Decreases *ATP which creates insulin resistance

- Increases triglycerides and LDL Cholesterol

- Increases blood pressure

- Increases the risk of heart disease

- Increases levels of uric acid

- Increases the risk of arterial plaque

- Can cause cavities as sugar metabolizes into acid

- When HFCS is ingested, the liver produces more fat than normal

- It makes the brain believe that you are still hungry

Statistics and Facts

- New cases of diabetes and pre-diabetes have increased 90% over the last 10-15 years

- Diabetes affects 1 in 4 Americans

- The use of HFCS in the diet increased 10,600% from 1970 to 2005 (USDA report)

- The increase of Type II Diabetes and HFCS has grown in parallel since the 1980's in the US alone

- Diabetes deaths in 1980 were 34,851 VS 73,138 in 2004

- A study in Switzerland links pancreatic cancer with the use of artificial sweeteners and HFCS

Artificial colors and flavors

- Created with petrochemicals and tar which cause cancer

- May cause learning disabilities

- In high amounts causes violent behavior

- It has been proven to cause male infertility

- These dyes can cause itching, migraines, headaches, acne and alteration of the nervous system

- Cause allergies and in some cases even death

- Green # 3 is linked to Bladder Cancer

- Yellow No. 5 causes allergic reactions, asthma attacks and several studies show that it causes thyroid tumors

- Red # 40 causes reactions such as aggressive behavior, shouting, kicking, nervousness, dizziness and hyperactivity

- Yellow # 2 is linked to Attention Deficit Hyperactivity Disorder or ADHD, in scientific studies

- Red # 2 is a carcinogenic and is no longer used in foods for many years but it can be used in cosmetics, medicines and some vaccines. Read the labels and stay away from them

Artificial Sugars

- They are Excitotoxins

- May increase obesity levels

- Can cause changes in metabolism

- May cause severe headaches or migraines

- Studies indicate that Aspartame can help produce cancerous tumors, leukemia, memory loss, Multiple Sclerosis, Parkinson's symptoms and premature death.

- Reduces levels of the hormone Serotonin

- More than 5,000 foods contain Aspartame. Read the labels

- The FDA denied approval of Aspartame for 8 years but it was finally approved by a government authority in 1981

- Can cause enlargement of the liver and kidneys

- Reports indicate that it reduces the Thymus Gland which is responsible for helping the immune system

- These are very similar to MSG

Foods to Avoid

- Processed Pork Products such as: Pepperoni, Salami, Bologna, Sausage, Bacon, Ham, Sausage

- Fried foods with hydrogenated oil or vegetable oil high in Omega 6

- Fish high in mercury such as: Swordfish, Shark, King Mackerel, Tilefish, Dolphin (Mahi-Mahi)

- Anything made with white processed flour

- Microwave frozen meals

- Doughnuts, corn chips, junk food in general

- Sodas, bottled pasteurized juices

- Cereals with all kinds of artificial colors made with GMO corn. If the package doesn't say non-GMO, it has GMO's

- Cow's milk

- GMO "foods" like fish, corn, soy, alfalfa, papaya, canola oil and zucchini. The labels won't tell you thanks to Congress, Monsanto and the large food companies.

Essential Foods

- Water (7-8 glasses a day). Add lemon to at least 1 cup per day

- Fruits such as apples, mango, avocado, figs, bananas, pears, melons, pineapple, orange, kiwi, lemons and all the berries

- Vegetables such as onions, broccoli, garlic, ginger, cucumber, celery, carrots, cauliflower, cabbage, artichoke and kale

- Beans, almonds, walnuts, Brazil nuts

- Fish with low or no mercury

- Juices and smoothies – Homemade of course

- Flaxseed, Omega 3, Wheat germ, chia seeds, fiber foods

- Green salads

- Water with lemon. Some people may be sensitive to lemon and develop skin stains or spots, if you do, just reduce the amount

- A glass of water with a pinch of baking soda each day. This elevates the water pH level and hence alkalizes the blood.

- Alkaline foods. I explain this in more detail in the cancer chapter

IMPORTANCE OF SUPPLEMENTS

- Vitamin C

- Vitamin D3

- Vitamin E

- B Complex

- Multi-vitamins

- Fiber

- Omega 3

Vitamin C

- Awesome Healing Powers
- Super anti-oxidant when taken in large amounts at saturation.
- Protects against immune system deficiencies
- Helps prevent cardiovascular disease, stroke, cancer and eye diseases
- Helps reduce wrinkles if natural forms are applied in the form of fruits and vegetables (organic is preferable)
- Reduces stress and helps with the flu and inflammation
- Helps to grow, build and repair body tissues
- It is an antioxidant that protects against free radical damage
- There are several forms of vitamin C including:
  - Ascorbic Acid (promotes acidity and can irritate the stomach, lasts up to 4 hours in the body, 25% is absorbed)
  - Sodium Ascorbate (Promotes alkalinity, it's stomach friendly, remains up to 14 hours, 95% is absorbed)

- Found in the following foods:

  Citrus fruits, red and green peppers, **strawberries**, tomatoes, **broccoli**, white and sweet potatoes, **melon**, papaya, mango, watermelon, blackberry, pineapple, blueberries, nectarine, **grapefruit, kiwi** and others

Vitamin D3

- When taken with vitamin C the body absorbs it better
- Keeps calcium levels balanced in the blood
- Helps maintain the immune system
- Plays an important role in insulin secretion
- Helps regulate blood pressure
- Helps prevent breast and prostate cancer
- Studies indicate that it plays a key role in the prevention of the following diseases: osteoporosis, cancer, Alzheimer's, hypertension, diabetes, arthritis, Multiple Sclerosis
- Sun blockers inhibit the skin from producing vitamin D
- Sunlight is the only reliable way to generate vitamin-D
- A person would need to drink 10 glasses of raw milk each day to get the minimum levels of vitamin D. More on this in the milk chapter
- Chronic vitamin D deficiency is misdiagnosed as Fibromyalgia because the symptoms are very similar
- Vitamin D deficiency can cause Schizophrenia
- The rest of the world uses Vitamin D to treat Psoriasis
- Vitamin D is 800% more effective than the flu vaccine, according to a study published in the American Journal of Clinical Nutrition

Vitamin E

- Antioxidant that neutralizes free radicals

- Protects cell membranes

- Maintains healthy skin, heart, nerves, muscles and red blood cells

- Reduces aging of cells

- Prevents abnormal blood clotting

- inhibits or prevents the growth of skin cancer (Melanoma)

- If taken with Vitamin A protects the lungs from pollutants, nervous system and retina as well as heart disease

- Reduces the risk of Alzheimer's, Parkinson's, asthma, rheumatoid arthritis and cataracts when taken in large quantities (1,000 IU) with Vitamin C (20,000 mg)

B Complex Vitamins

- B1 or Thiamin - Helps the nervous system, energy production, physical strength. Deficiency causes beriberi. It acts as a natural repellent
- B2 or Riboflavin - For the health of the skin. Deficiency of this vitamin can cause extreme sun sensitivity, dermatitis and cracked / dry lips
- B3 or Niacin - Essential for mental health, memory loss, mental confusion and depression
- B5 or Pantothenic Acid - Metabolizes proteins, carbohydrates and fats
- B6 or Pyridoxine - Helps produce red blood cells and aids with cardiovascular health. Keeps healthy skin
- B7 or Biotin - Essential for growing babies. In adults it is essential for the synthesis of fatty acids and blood sugar level. Helps strengthen hair. It is being studied for the treatment of diabetes
- B9 or Folic Acid - Can prevent heart disease and anemia. Maintains and repairs cells, helps metabolize amino acids and DNA synthesis. Helps form red & white blood cells
- B12 or Cobalamin - Essential for anemia because it helps with the production of red blood cells. It can reverse anemia better than iron. Essential to maintain a healthy nervous system. Aids in the production of DNA and regulates the formation of red blood cells. Increases energy levels. Very good for those suffering from high cholesterol or heart disease. The best form is Methyl Cobalamin

Multi-Vitamins

- Essential for overall health because they contain vitamins and minerals that the body needs daily such as zinc, copper, manganese and others

- Many are made with synthetic ingredients and only a small percentage is absorbed

- Look for vitamins without artificial colors or flavors

- Make sure they are food-based and non-GMO

- Do not buy the cheapest. Read the ingredients. When it comes to vitamins, the cheapest are the worst kind

- Look for those that are specific for men, women or seniors

- Don't believe the myth that says "Foods contain all the vitamins and minerals you need". This may be true but the levels are too low

- The more you eat the more vitamins you need because, eating a lot of food means burning a lot of food and more free radicals are produced

- They allow your body to grow and develop as well as help maintain healthy cells throughout your body

Fiber

- Reduces the glycemic effect of meals

- It can lower cholesterol, triglycerides and LDL

- May help prevent ulcers, diabetes, cancer, heart disease and kidney stones

- Relieves hemorrhoids and constipation

- Keeps weight under control

- Accelerates the movement of food through the colon

- Reduces heart attacks, strokes and tachycardia

- Reduces arterial plaque growth and controls blood clots

- Helps reduce blood pressure

- Reduces cell inflammation

- Studies indicate that it relieves pain in patients with rheumatoid arthritis

- Studies are being conducted for treatment of ADD, ADHD and Autism

  Sources: Fruits, vegetables, grains, whole grains, flaxseed, Chia seeds and others

DISEASES

- Diabetes

- Heart Disease

- Cancer

- Alzheimer's

- Obesity

DIABETES

I can write an entire book about diabetes and I eventually will in the near future. I researched a lot information about diabetes because of the history of this disease in my house. In the mean time, I want to share with you some of my research in this summarized chapter. This subject affects millions of people around the world and kills about 76,000 people each year in the United States alone, making it the number 7 cause of death in the US. Currently in the United States there are about 100 million people who are diagnosed as pre-diabetic. This means that if these people don't make any changes in their life style and eating habits, the number of deaths related to this disease will be greater in the years to come. The biggest problem is that many of these pre-diabetic cases are children. A great majority of these cases can be avoided with proper nutrition, diet and exercise. This is sad because the foods these kids eat are purchased by parents who unknowingly are causing a lot of suffering to their kids and themselves. Later in this chapter you will learn which foods increase the chances of getting diabetes and which foods could reduce glucose levels which may reverse some cases of diabetes. You will also learn how to prevent diabetes and some of the statistics related to this terrible disease. Most people don't know that diabetes is a slow killer that little by little reduces eye vision until total blindness and many patients lose their limbs in the form of medical amputations due to poor circulation.

As I indicated earlier, my mother died of type II diabetes. That is why this topic is very close to me and my siblings in particular. According to experts, this disease is caused primarily by poor diet based on refined carbohydrates, sugars and others which I will explain in more detail later. Diabetes is one of those diseases that can be easily avoided but the person must have the desire and commitment to do so. There are two types of diabetes.

Type 1 diabetes mellitus is less common than type 2 and is more common in young people. The number of people with type 1 diabetes is approximately 5% of the overall disease statistics. People suffering from this type of diabetes produce little or no insulin and therefore they must supplement it with daily insulin. This is why type 1 diabetes is also known as insulin dependent diabetes. According to Mayo Clinic, the exact cause of type 1 diabetes is unknown. However, some experts believe it is caused by childhood vaccines. Doctor J. Classen who is an expert immunologist discovered this and other illnesses associated with metabolic syndrome. Since vaccines tend to over stimulate the immune system, they may inhibit the production of insulin which results in the development of type 1 diabetes. In some cases, vaccines increase the production of too much insulin which may eventually cause type 2 Diabetes. As I said before, every human body is different and hence the reason vaccines don't affect every person the same way.

Type 2 Diabetes is a chronic condition that affects how the body metabolizes sugar or glucose which is the body's main source of energy. According to the American Diabetes Association (ADA), in type 2 diabetes, your body doesn't use insulin properly. This is called insulin resistance. Basically the pancreas makes extra insulin whenever it senses a spike in glucose in your blood. Your pancreas is supposed to excrete insulin whenever your glucose intake is too high. So when you eat a meal high in sugar or refined carbohydrates or even just a large meal, the pancreas knows what to do and it automatically excretes the right amount of insulin to balance the glucose levels. The problem is when the pancreas has to do this too many times a day, weeks or months, the pancreas can't keep up with the overload and can't make enough insulin to keep your blood glucose levels normal. This causes insulin resistance and what we know today as type 2 diabetes. According to the ADA and Mayo clinic, there is no cure for diabetes. However, many doctors, nutritionists and scientists disagree. Food plays a big role in either causing or reversing many diseases. Diabetes is not an exception to this. Poor diet is perhaps the number 1 cause of type 2 diabetes and while many institutions don't believe that this disease can actually be prevented or even reversed, there are many cases that prove otherwise. A poor diet high in sugar is the precursor of pre-diabetes and diabetes. What most people don't know is that many foods contain large amounts of sugar in the form of carbohydrates. The amount of sugar contained in carbohydrates and other foods is measured by something called the Glycemic Index or GI. This measures how a carbohydrate-containing food raises blood glucose. A food with a high GI will raise the blood glucose more rapidly than a food with a medium or low GI. So, one of the keys to reducing blood glucose levels is to adopt a diet containing low GI foods. If you are pre-diabetic some experts recommend a ratio equal to 60% low GI foods and 35% med GI foods and 5% high GI foods. If you already have been diagnosed with type 2 diabetes, you should follow a ratio equal to 70%-75% low GI and 25%-30% med GI foods and no high GI foods at all. Later in this chapter I will give you the list of foods with low, medium and high GI levels for you to plan your food intake. Another key to reducing blood glucose levels is to increase your fiber intake. Most people don't eat a balanced diet rich in fiber. These people are making a costly mistake because fiber is essential for preventing many diseases including type 2 diabetes. Foods with high GI levels cause a rapid spike in blood glucose and they eventually cause glucose to begin to build in the blood instead of going into the cells. This causes the cells to starve for energy. This also causes long term complications such as poor eye sight, kidney, nerve problems and heart disease. Did you know that white bread has a very high glycemic index number and the body converts it to glucose (sugar) as quickly as white sugar? White bread has a GI equal to 71 while white pasta has a GI of 92. So the more white bread and pasta you eat the more glucose your body coverts and the more insulin your pancreas excretes. The more high GI foods you eat the faster you will develop type 2 diabetes. What do you prefer, control the disease with potentially dangerous drugs or prevent the disease in the first place? I think the choice is clear. Trust me, this disease is no joke and as I mentioned at the beginning of this book I saw my own mother suffer with this disease until the day she died. If I only knew what I know today, I probably could've saved her life or at least extend it by many years.

In the next few pages I give you a summarized version of this disease, its statistics, how to prevent it and the different GI foods to eat and to avoid.

A note from the author: By law I cannot guarantee you anything but it is very possible that if you follow these points for two consecutive months, you may cure type 2 diabetes. I know it's hard but try it for at least two weeks and see what happens. Let your doctor know what you want to do before making drastic changes to your diet and life style. You will be surprised of the results.

Diabetes summary

- Diabetes is the #7 cause of death in the United States with approximately 76,000 deaths per year
- 25.8 Million people in the US have diabetes
- 100 Million people are pre-diabetic
- 99% of type 2 diabetes can be reversible if drastic measures are taken
- The American Diabetes Association was founded in 1940 but the diabetes rates are much higher today than ever before. What is the ADA doing? Not much in my opinion
- Diabetes is not in the top 20 causes of death in the world but it is the #7 in the United States. Americans are addicted to sugar
- Diabetes cause heart complications, high blood pressure, blindness, kidney disease, amputations and others
- More than half of the leg amputations are done to diabetes patients. This is a fact
- Reduces the quality of life mainly due to the use of prescription medicines
- Diabetes medicines can cause serious damage to the liver, kidneys and heart as well as strokes and even death as I explained earlier with the drug Avandia
- Rezulin was pulled from the market 6 months after Europe pulled it. This diabetes drug killed about 10,000 people and left about 100,000 people injured with liver damage.
- The World Health Organization predicts that the number of diabetes deaths will increase by 2/3 between 2008 and 2030. This is really bad news

- 90% of diabetics in the world have type 2 diabetes and this is the result of poor diet, lack of exercise and obesity
- Diabetes increases the risk of heart attacks and strokes
- 68% of diabetics die from heart complications and strokes. My mother died of heart complications and had a few minor strokes 6 months prior to her death
- After 10 years with diabetes, 2% become blind and 10% have severe eye sight impediment
- Diabetes is the highest cause of severe kidney disease
- The Glycemic Index in food is extremely important in the fight against diabetes or the prevention of this disease
- There are low, medium and high Glycemic Index numbers. The lower the number the better for diabetics
- White bread, pasta, pastries, bagels, doughnuts, waffles and pancakes are among the foods with the highest GI number
- Green vegetables, most fruits and nuts are among the foods with the lowest GI
- Drinking a lot of water will help you reduce the effects of high GI foods. Add some lemon to raise the pH level
- Water also helps the kidneys work better

How to Prevent Diabetes*

*This statement has not been evaluated by the FDA

- Lose weight with good nutrition and exercise
- Eat a diet low in fat and sugar
- Check blood pressure every so often
- Eliminate High Fructose Corn Syrup
- Reduce or eliminate processed white flour
- Reduce or eliminate foods & fruits with high Glycemic Index
- Eat foods high in fiber (very important)
- Eat green vegetables every day. They have low Glycemic Index
- Take half your weight in ounces of water every day
- Limit your sodium intake, alcohol and caffeine
- Cook with coconut oil
- Eliminate artificial sweeteners. Use Stevia
- Do not eat anything with trans fats or hydrogenated oil
- Avoid fast foods and instant microwavable foods
- Take one or two cups of Green Tea daily without sugar
- Eat fruits and vegetables rich in anti-oxidants and low GI
- Do not eat white rice, pasta, donuts, watermelon, corn flakes, Rice Krispies, Cheerios, saltine crackers, chips, instant rice, white bread, bagel, waffles and white flour pancakes.
- Eliminate all dairy products and meats

Foods with high Glycemic Index

- Parsnips (97)*

- Pasta (92)

- Baked potato (85)

- Instant Potato (83)

- Corn cakes (83)

- Rice Krispies (82)

- Crackers (81)

- wafer cookies (77)

- Donuts (76)

- Waffles (76)

- Hash Browns (75)

- Corn chips (74)

- White bread (71)

- Watermelon (72)

- Graham crackers (71)

*The number in parenthesis denotes the Glycemic number of each food listed. The higher the number the more you should avoid it.

Foods with medium Glycemic Index

- Mashed potatoes (70)
- Crushed wheat (69)
- Taco flour (68)
- Croissant (67)
- Angel Cake (67)
- Pineapple (66)
- White Sugar (65)
- Macaroni and cheese (64)
- Raisins (64)
- Biscuits (64)
- Muffins (62)
- Ice cream (61)
- Hamburger bun (61)
- Cheese pizza (61)
- White rice (58)
- Mango (56)
- Popcorn (55)
- Spaghetti (55)
- Fruit Cocktail (55)

Foods with low Glycemic Index

- Low fat plain yogurt
- Peanuts, almonds
- Artichoke
- Asparagus
- Broccoli, cauliflower
- Celery, Carrots
- Cucumber
- Eggplant
- Peas
- Lettuce
- All peppers
- Spinach
- Tomato, Zuccini
- cherries
- Barley
- Grapefruit, lemon, orange
- Lentils
- Apples, pears

HEART DISEASE

This should be one of the biggest concerns for everyone since heart disease is the number one killer in the United States and the world. In the United States alone, about 2,500 people die each day from heart related complications. It is by far the biggest killer of all diseases. Many people don't know this, and know it they must, because they are killing themselves with their dietary choices without even knowing it. It is believed that the wrong foods are the number 1 cause of heart disease accounting for about 85% of the cases. Processed foods, animal saturated fat including all meats, cow's milk, cheese and fried junk food are the biggest contributors to heart disease.

A recent study led by researches from Harvard School of Public Health and Cambridge Health Alliance, showed that a Mediterranean-style diet was associated with lower risk of cardiovascular disease (CVD). A diet rich in fish, nuts, olive oil, vegetables and fruits have been shown in other previous studies to reduce the risk of CVD. Such is the case of the Lyon Diet Heart Study as described in the book "Ultra Prevention" by doctors Mark Hyman and Mark Liponis. In this book they noted how a 46 month study on the heart looked at 600 men and women who had suffered a heart attack and survived. Some of these people were told to eat a Mediterranean diet while the rest were told to eat the American Heart Association heart disease, prevention and cholesterol lowering diet. The Mediterranean diet included fat from foods such as fish, olive oil, lots of fruits and vegetables, beans, nuts, seeds, eggs and some wine. It also had much higher portions of fiber than the American Heart Association diet. It also included high amounts of Omega 3 fatty acids. The results were amazing. The people eating the Mediterranean diet had 50% to 70% fewer second heart attacks than the other group. This result was so significant that the American Heart Association guidelines for a healthy heart had to be revised. They even had to stop the study early because too many people eating the American Heart Association diet were dying from heart attack. So, the main thing to learn from this study is that, not all fats are created equal. Fats from fish, nuts, avocado, olive oil and seeds are much healthier than saturated fats, Omega

6 and trans fats or hydrogenated oils. If you eat too much of these fats you will clog your arteries and eventually develop heart disease. On the other hand, if you eat a diet rich in good fats, you will prevent a heart attack, have healthier nails and even reverse the signs of depression. Some of this information is common sense but unfortunately most people don't know this and are unknowingly causing themselves harm with their dietary choices. The sad thing is that many people shrug of this type of information and don't pay attention to books like this until it is too late. Please remember that heart disease doesn't happen over night; it builds up over a long period of time. An artery could take decades to clog; the bad news is... your body doesn't tell you when that artery is completely clogged to the point that one afternoon meal could be your last meal. The good news is.... You can reverse heart disease if you make changes to your diet NOW, not later. Don't be part of these terrible statistics. Also, don't think that this could only happen to you until you are 65 or 70 years young. Heart disease is happening at a much earlier age today than ever before. There are people in their early 40's having a heart attack; that's pretty scary if you ask me. I was heading that way and that's the main reason I changed my way of eating.

Another scary part of heart disease is strokes and aneurysms. As defined by WebMD.com a brain aneurysm is a bulging weak area in the wall of the artery that supplies blood to the brain. The problem is that this causes no symptoms and happens unexpectedly. Sometimes an aneurysm ruptures and spreads blood into the skull causing a stroke. Depending on how bad the hemorrhage is, this can cause permanent brain damage or death. No matter how you look at heart disease, it is bad news and it will kill you unless you make changes to your diet, reduce stress levels, exercise and lose weight. There are several ways to test your heart health. I don't recommend X-Rays or CT scans due to the cumulative effect of radiation. Other tests that are safer or non invasive are MRI's, Stress Test, Electrocardiogram and Echocardiogram (Transthoracic, Stress). You need to talk to your cardiologist and ask him/her for the best test for you based on the symptoms. Don't forget to remind your doctor about the dangers of x-rays and CT scans and remember that it is your body and the final decision is yours.

Symptoms of Coronary Artery Disease

This is a well known disease and the most common symptom is angina or chest pain. This can be mistaken for a heartburn because the symptoms are similar so be careful if you keep having pressure on the chest, burning, squeezing, heaviness and overall discomfort on the chest area. Other symptoms include sweating, nausea, weakness or dizziness, irregular and faster than normal heartbeats and shortness of breath.

Symptoms of a Heart Attack

A heart attack is also known as the silent killer or silent myocardial infarction because some people have a heart attack without having any symptoms at all. This happens more often on people with diabetes. If you think you're having a heart attack, call 911 right away because every second counts.

The most common symptoms are: Discomfort; pain in the chest, arm or below the breastbone; pain radiating to the back, jaw, arm or throat; fullness, indigestion like a heartburn feeling; extreme weakness, anxiety or shortness of breath and rapid and irregular beats.

How to prevent heart disease*
*This statement has not been evaluated by the FDA

This is the part that most people don't want to hear about because it involves making changes to their dietary choices. Heart disease doesn't happen overnight and hence reversing it will not happen overnight. It takes commitment, good will and determination. As I mentioned before, heart disease kills more people than any other disease and that's the reason you need to get serious about prevention. According to Mayo Clinic you can avoid heart problems by adopting a healthy life style. Below are 6 prevention tips to help you avoid this disease.

Stop smoking

This is the most significant risk factor for developing heart disease. The chemicals in tobacco can damage the heart and blood vessels, causing narrowing of the arteries also known as atherosclerosis. Women who smoke and take birth control pills are at greater risk because both of these increase the risk of blood clots.

Exercise

This is a no brainer. The heart is a muscle and therefore it needs to be exercised to be healthy. When you exercise for 30 to 45 minutes each day of the week your heart will thank you. Physical activity helps you control your weight and will help you reduce the risk of other conditions such as diabetes, high blood pressure and high cholesterol to name a few. You don't even have to engage in strenuous physical activities, you can start by walking every day and gradually increase your activity until your body asks for more. Trust me, it will become a habit and you will feel bad when you don't do it. For me, exercise is a must even if it's a few push-ups or pull-ups each day. So get off the couch and start today. Put the TV remote aside and get on it NOW.

Heart Healthy Diet

I don't think I have to get on too many details on this subject as this should be obvious to most people. A diet rich in fruits, vegetables and whole grains will protect your heart and may prevent a heart attack as explained earlier with the Mediterranean diet. Try to limit your intake of saturated fats (no more than 10% of daily calories) and completely avoid hydrogenated oils or Trans fats. Saturated fats are those from red meats and dairy products. Trans fats are the most dangerous ones and they are found in deep fried fast foods, bakery products, processed snacks, crackers and margarines. Do not cut all fats from your diet though; some fats are good for you and essential to your life. Healthy fats include fish oils, nuts, olives, olive oil and avocado. If you want to avoid heart disease, diabetes and cancer and keep out of the horrible death statistics, eat 8-10 servings of fruits and vegetables, drink in moderation, eat fish 2-3 times per week, avoid Trans fats and consume the right fats. It is that simple. Don't fall into the pharmaceutical trap. Your body wasn't designed to take medicines. Enjoy life to its fullest. You owe it to your family and yourself.

Keep your weight on check

As you may already know, two thirds of Americans are overweight. Your chances of heart disease, high blood pressure, high cholesterol and diabetes increase when you have excess weight around your middle area. One rule of thumb to consider if you want to know if you are overweight is to measure your waist line. For men, it should be less than 40 inches while women should have no more than 35 inches. Small amounts of weight loss are beneficial since a 5-10% can decrease blood pressure, cholesterol levels and reduce the risk of diabetes.

The last two prevention tips are regular health screenings and getting plenty of sleep. These two are just as important as the other four. Regular screenings will help you know where you are and will serve as a baseline for you to start making changes to your diet and lifestyle. Knowing what your health looks like with blood test screenings should motivate you to change your life for a better health future. Remember, you are in this world for a reason so live life like it's meant to be lived. Enjoy it and live with passion.

Heart Disease Summary

- It is the # 1 cause of death in the USA. One in two Americans die each year

- Every 34 seconds a person dies of a heart attack in the USA

- More than 2,500 people die each day in the USA. This is huge and everyone should be concerned about it

- Today, over 5,000 people get a heart surgery at a cost of $50 billion dollars a year

- Smoking accelerates the progression of atherosclerosis which is the precursor of heart disease

- High cholesterol is not the only measure of heart disease. There are 16 others including C-Reactive Protein or CRP, Homocysteine, hypertension, high triglycerides and low HDL

- Countries with fewer heart attack deaths are Japan, France, Spain and Switzerland

- Eliminate Trans fats or hydrogenated oils and Omega 6 fats

- Choose foods low in saturated fat and polyunsaturated fat

- Do aerobic exercise at least 3 times a week

- Cut down on fatty meats such as beef and pork

- Do not eat processed meats (pepperoni, sausage, salami, bacon and ham)

- Reduce Blood Pressure

- Lose weight without diets or drugs. Just go out and move

- Reduce Stress, Increase fiber and vegetables in your diet

- Prevent and control diabetes

- Do not smoke

- If you drink liquor, do not take more than one drink per day

- Check the levels of Homocysteine, C-Reactive protein, triglycerides, LDL and glucose

- Maintain optimal levels of vitamin D and vitamin K

- Take CO-Q10 especially if you take cholesterol drugs

- Eat fish oils

- Increase intake of Omega 3 (EPA, DHA) and Omega 9 (avocado, olive oil, nuts)

CANCER

Cancer is a multi-billion dollar industry and today is almost impossible for government agencies like the FDA, CDC and the AMA to accept the fact that cancer can be cured without the use of the only approved drugs for this disease such as chemotherapy and radiation. Many people don't know there are clinics and doctors in the United States and around the world that are curing cancer using alternative medicines, good diet and natural methods based on good nutrition. The cancer industry is so powerful that each time a doctor has provided a different therapy to treat or cure cancer other than chemotherapy and radiation; they have been ridiculed and even sued by the American Cancer Society (ACS) or the FDA. Such is the case of Dr. Burzynski who has had to endure attacks from the FDA, the ACS and the board of oncologists in Texas. These entities have taken this doctor to court several times. The only thing that this doctor has done is cure hundreds or thousands of patients from different types of cancer over the past 20 years. Dr. Burzynski invented a drug (Anti-neoplastons) that cures cancer but has no side effects. He receives no funding from the government or the ACS. To learn more about this doctor I recommend you to watch the documentary "Dr Burzynski, the Movie". The only thing I warn you is that after seeing this film you will be completely shocked and speechless when you learn about the corruption and conspiracy that exists to silence and weaken any doctor, scientist or nutritionist who tries to cure cancer. I know right now you're probably thinking that something like this cannot be happening in the 21st century here in the land of the free, the beautiful United States of America. How can that be? Impossible, right? Wrong. It has been happening every day for many decades.

How can it be that there are cures for cancer but these entities want to silence these doctors instead of spreading the good news that cancer can be cured? As I said before, the cancer industry is huge and powerful. Now think about this, if these cures that exist had the government backing, the FDA helping and especially national and international news talking about it every day, what do you think will happen to these agencies and the hundreds of nonprofit cancer organizations? Obviously they would have to close their doors because cancer would be cured. The same thing will happen to the thousands of cancer clinics, oncologists, radiology technicians, nurses, mammography clinics and buses, walks and marathons which bring a lot of money to the cities and companies that sponsor this cause, etc. etc. Practically it would be a financial collapse of large magnitudes and governments know this. For this reason, the cure from big Pharma and the FDA will most likely never happen in the next 50 years or more. There is a lot of corruption out there. Please note that the president of the American Cancer Society has a salary of over two million dollars. Don't you think this is unfair? This society is a non-profit agency and receives millions of dollars from the government (your taxes), donations from companies and people like you and I. These donations are supposed to be used for the continued research of the cure. But how long do we have to wait for the cure? This company was founded in 1913 with the mission to cure cancer. Don't you think that 100 years is a long time? How can they keep lying to the world that there is still no cure for cancer when history says otherwise? The Gerson Institute in California and Mexico, Dr. Gonzalez in New York, Dr. Burzynski in Texas, Canyon Ranch Health Resort, The Hippocrates Health Institute in West Palm Beach and others have been curing cancer for a long time. The only reason we don't know about these is because these doctors and institutions are prohibited by federal law to disclose or publish that they are curing cancer with treatments or medications that are not approved by the FDA.

If a doctor or scientist has a drug or therapy that cures cancer and that doctor comes out on the news and says he's curing cancer using drugs or treatments that are not approved by the FDA, that doctor can go to jail for many years because it is a federal crime to say that a drug or therapy other than those approved by the FDA can cure cancer. Even if that drug cures 100% of the patients. If it's not approved by the FDA, that doctor can go to federal prison for more than 30 years. Hard to believe, but true. Any doctor or scientist who speaks negatively about the conventional medicines such as chemotherapy or radiation is dismissed or ridiculed by the greatest authorities of the medical system. Such is the case of Dr. Julian Nicholas who studied at Oxford University and Mayo Clinic and who was an employee of the FDA in 2009. In June 2009, this doctor wrote a letter to the medical directors of the FDA to put a warning to caution patients of the dangers of radiation from CT scans. In this letter, Dr. Nicholas said that this procedure may cause abdominal cancer and leukemia. Possibly not caused at the time of the examination, but may eventually cause cancer.. Dr. Nicholas was dismissed from his job by the FDA and is now teaching at a university. This is the kind of abuse that exists and nobody talks about it. If you believe that none of this can be true, or that I made it up, please do your own research in other books and journals, or check the history of cancer, or other reliable sources. The internet is not always the best source, but if that's the only source available at your finger tips, you can visit reputable sites that have reliable and trustworthy information about this subject.

The cure for cancer is at your fingertips but you have to have the courage and determination to do so. It is not easy but not impossible. There are several books about cancer cures. One is "Cancer can be cured" by the Franciscan Roman Father, Zago. There are many books like this. If you or a loved one has cancer, educate yourself, don't play heads or tails with an oncologist because it is very likely that he cannot give you even a 50% chance of getting cured with traditional treatments like chemotherapy and radiation. These methods are barbaric in my opinion and only have a long term success rate of 2%. You are the owner of your body and you have to decide what you want to do. If you prefer to follow the recommendation of your oncologist before trying alternative therapies, that is your choice, may God help you and I really hope you get better and get cured.

You may be wondering why radiation and chemotherapy are so bad? And why are they not effective? As I explained earlier, radiation causes cancer because it is cumulative and with each radiation therapy you receive your body is exposed to certain amounts, measured in millisieverts. The higher this number, the higher the possibility of creating other tumors. Ionizing radiation like X-rays, mammograms, CT scans and those use for cancer treatments, has sufficient energy to remove an electron from an atom or molecule. It is so strong that it damages DNA in the cells and these cells become so unstable that they experience very rapid, drastic changes and mutations which can cause cancer and eventual death of the cells in the area that has been irradiated. The reason it is believed that the radiation is not 100% effective, is because there are several types of cancer cells. The most aggressive cells are called Stem Cells, which only require a small cell to reproduce millions of new cells. The other cells are less aggressive and die relatively easy.

Did you know that the success of radiation and chemotherapy is measured with physical reduction of a tumor? Did you also know that more than half of the cells in a tumor are not aggressive? This is why Oncologists tell their patients (after treatment) that the tumor was reduced by 50% or X% and therefore the treatment is "working". What they don't tell you (perhaps because they don't know) is that the stem cells that resist treatment can reproduce within a few days or months after radiation. These stem cells are extremely aggressive and resist most of these barbaric therapies and feed on other cells that have been weakened by several reasons such as poor diet, the environment, stress and the effects of smoking. That's why the first thing a cancer patient should do is to change his or her diet dramatically and opt for a strict green vegetable based diet, certain fruits, green drinks like Green Super Foods and certain types of supplements. Eat a highly alkaline diet and reduce or avoid eating acidic foods or foods that are converted to acid ash inside your body. Don't confused acidic foods with acid tasting foods. For example, lemons and grapefruits are acid tasting fruits but they are highly alkaline and raise the pH level. I'm talking about foods that are metabolized to sugar and then converted to acid ash in your body, such as refined carbohydrates, white pasta, white rice, sugar and others. Refined carbohydrates are converted to palmitic acid which is then synthesize into what we know as triglycerides. A complete list is given in the alkaline and acid foods section in the next few pages. Another important combination that breaks cancer tumors is curcumin and black pepper which can be 1,000 times more effective than chemotherapy.

If you opt for radiation, I advise you to question your oncologist and ask if the clinic uses a new method called Focused Radiation. Also make sure that the applied radiation is the minimum amount necessary to irradiate the tumor. These machines have radiation controls for low or high levels. The higher the level, the higher the damage to your organs. And remember, your organs are the ones being damaged not theirs so don't be afraid to ask and demand more details of the potential side effects of this treatment. Good luck.

Milk

Every one of us has been told that milk is good for us. Got Milk? Remember the white mustache commercials? When you are asked - what are the two main benefits of drinking milk? Most likely, you will answer what 98% of the people answer, calcium, protein and vitamin D. Well, I am sorry to tell you that we have all been lied to or at least partially lied to. The reason is, they are not telling us the whole truth or at least they are not telling us the potential risks associated with drinking cow's milk. Milk is great for you, if you are a calf. Cow's milk has about 59 active hormones, saturated fat, cholesterol and many allergens that challenge the human body's immune system every time we drink this good tasting white liquid. Studies have found that milk has herbicides, dioxins, powerful antibiotics stronger than those given to humans, pesticides, blood, pus, feces, bacteria and viruses. The number one cause of death in the US and most developed countries is heart disease. Think about all the saturated fat, cholesterol and dairy that these countries consume with the help of milk. The milk industry makes us believe that milk is an essential food in our food supply.

Milk has a powerful hormone called insulin-like growth factor one or IGF-1. This hormone has been shown to be a key factor in the rapid growth and proliferation of prostate, colon and breast cancers. Other cancers may also be promoted by this hormone. This hormone may be important for calves not humans because it helps them grow faster and fatter. Monsanto invented a powerful injection that helps cows produce more milk than normal. This shot is called Posilac (or rbGH). This shot helps generate more IGF-1 in milk (up to 80% more). Unfortunately for you and I the FDA says that this IGF-1 is destroyed in the stomach and therefore we don't have to worry about anything. Common sense tells us that this claim by the FDA is ridiculous because this hormone makes the baby calf grow faster. If this hormone is destroyed in our stomachs then human digestion and absorption don't work at all do they?

Where do you think cows get the calcium for their BIG bones? From plants, of course. The plants they eat have large amounts of magnesium which is needed to properly absorb and use calcium. Cow's milk has very little traces of magnesium so the calcium in milk is useless to humans because most of that calcium cannot be absorbed by a human body. There is a reason why cows have 4 stomachs and humans only have one. Even though cow's milk has three times the calcium as human breast milk, it doesn't really matter because you need an equal amount of magnesium to be able to absorb and use calcium. To give you an idea, milk has enough magnesium to absorb about 11% of calcium. The countries with the highest rates of osteoporosis are also the countries with the highest consumption of cow's milk. Check the 12 year Harvard study on 78,000 nurses. Nurses with the highest consumption of milk per day had a significantly higher risk of hip fracture (45% increase). Milk is considered to be acidic in the pH table. In the next chapter I explain the dangers of eating foods that have a pH of less than 7. When you drink milk and other dairy products in a daily basis your body needs to alkalize the effects of this acid forming food. To do this the body gets the most alkalizing mineral in your body, CALCIUM, from your alkaline reserves inside your body or the alkalizing food you eat (which unfortunately is very little). If you don't have enough calcium reserves your body automatically goes to your bones to extract the calcium it needs to balance the acid from the milk. So, if you drink too much milk or consume too many dairy products, your bones will eventually become brittle and increase your risk of bone fractures. I hope you understand why the calcium from milk is not really that beneficial for humans?

Now, let's talk about the protein in milk. 80% of the protein found in milk is called Casein. This is a powerful binder or polymer and it is used to make plastics. Casein is also used to make glue for furniture and to hold the labels on most glass bottles. Casein is bad news as it creates lots of mucus, especially in infants and young children. So if you're an athlete don't eat pizza or any other diary food before your run or exercise routine. Pasteurization of milk kills all bacteria (good and bad). While it sounds good to kill the bacteria, this actually creates another problem in milk. There are several enzymes in milk; one of these enzymes is needed for proper absorption and processing of casein. The problem is – pasteurization kills this enzyme and the body cannot properly process casein. When this happens casein finds its way into weak cells and binds and clogs cells and ducts that are designed to flow freely like milk ducts in women breasts. The accumulation of this binding agent may cause fungus or small tumors on the breast. If nothing is done to dissolve this fungus, over the years, it can grow slowly until it creates a tumor big enough to be detected by cancer detection methods. Homogenization of milk is also bad news because it helps break up large fat molecules into small ones. These small fat molecules get into the bloodstream which helps fat-borne toxins to get into the organs. Large fat molecules cannot enter the intestinal wall into the bloodstream so if you like cow's milk, try to find raw milk. Unfortunately for you, the FDA banned raw milk which is better than the regular milk you are allowed to buy at the supermarkets. That's the FDA for you.

Cow's milk has also been connected to type 1 diabetes. The American Academy of Pediatrics (AAP) issued the following warning, "Early exposure of infants to cow's milk protein may be an important factor in the initiation of the beta cell (insulin-producing cells of the pancreas) destructive process in some individuals." Exposure to cow's milk protein early in life, sometimes causes the protein to enter the bloodstream where antibodies are made by the immune system. These antibodies also attack the insulin-producing cells of the pancreas. So, if the AAP is worried about infants for the first several months of life or prior to age one, why aren't they worried about age 2, 3, 4, etc.? they should be worried about all ages because children love ice cream, butter, cheese and other dairy products that help with the initiation of the beta cell. No wonder why type 1 diabetes is mostly found in people of young age. Type 2 diabetes is a different animal but milk may also help with this type of diabetes. A protein found in milk called Lactalbumin has been identified as a key factor in diabetes and one of the major reasons for the AAP to issue the statement mentioned above. I don't know about you but if I knew a product has been shown to weaken the pancreas which is the organ that excretes insulin to balance glucose levels, I'm not giving that product to my children. If you can't eliminate it, at least reduce it slowly.

Did you know that the FDA and the USDA allows commercial milk to have about 750,000 somatic cells, also known as pus, and 20,000 live bacteria for every 1 cubic centimeter? This is equivalent to 20 million live bacteria and 750 million pus cells per liter. Got pus?

The British medical journal Lancet reported that there is a close relationship between dairy consumption and Multiple Sclerosis or MS. Also, back in

2001 the journal of immunology linked MS to milk consumption. Doctor Michael Dosch, MD, also linked MS with milk protein. Him and his team of researchers found a close link between type 1 diabetes and MS. They believe these diseases are actually the same. Two thirds of MS victims are women and who do you think are mostly targeted by the dairy industry and its powerful marketing? Women. Cheese is mostly consumed by women and with the scare tactics of the dairy industry related to the misinformation on osteoporosis, they also fall for the milk consumption trap.

Dairy foods were the most recalled foods in the US between 1993 and 1998, mainly due to bacterial contamination such as salmonella, listeria and E. coli. These come from animal waste. They also contained viruses known to cause lymphoma and leukemia-like diseases. In the United States and worldwide, leukemia is more common in people that consume high amounts of dairy products. Multiple studies have shown that dairy farmers have an increase incidence of leukemia. Pasteurization kills many types of bacteria but some of it doesn't get killed. There is also a concern that pasteurization may break viruses into small fragments which can actually become more dangerous.

With all the evidence on the dangers of milk consumption, I have chosen to remove milk and other dairy products from my grocery shopping list. I occasionally eat a slice of pizza or a scoop of ice cream but I make sure it is a veggie pizza so I can reap the alkalizing benefits of the vegetables. I also drink alkaline water daily so a slice of pizza every once in a while won't cause me any long term damage. I rather prevent diseases from entering my house by eating well and avoiding the wrong foods. We only drink almond and rice milk at home and I hope you reduce your cow's milk consumption slowly but surely. There is a lot more information on the dangers of milk but as I said before, this book is summarized to make sure you read the book from cover to cover.

Mammography

Breast cancer is the number one cause of cancer deaths in women between the ages of 42-56 years in the US. One in eight women is diagnosed with breast cancer in the US; but yet only one in twenty Asian women are diagnosed with this type of cancer. It is believed that the reason may be in the differences in their diet. Asian women eat more fiber and foods with high nutritional value. They also drink tea all day and eat more soy which has been proven to lower the effects of estrogen and prevent breast cancer.

In an interview with actress and author Suzanne Somers, the well known neurosurgeon Dr. Russell Blaylock, told Mrs. Somers that if he were a woman he would never have a mammogram. He explains that a woman who has one mammogram each year for 10 consecutive years, has a 20% to 30% higher chance of developing breast cancer by the cumulative effects of radiation. Mike Adams, editor of the health news website Naturalnews.com explains in several articles and supported by scientific studies that exposure to radiation in the US has increased over 600% in the last 30 years. Most of this increase comes from patients exposed to radiation from medical equipment such as CT scans and mammograms.

The problem with this is that most people don't know that ionizing radiation from these procedures is extremely dangerous because of their cumulative effect as previously explained. Most patients and unfortunately many doctors don't know that only one exposure to a CT scan is equivalent to as much as four hundred X-rays. Yes, 400.

A study published in the New England Journal of Medicine in 2007 found that survivors of the atomic bombs dropped on Japan in 1945 during World War II, still face a significant increase in cancer risk today. These cases of radiation are equivalent to just 2 or 3 CT scans. Only two CT scans may be the same as been just a few miles from the explosion of an atomic bomb; this is a scientific fact.

Imagine then the risks that are exposed to those who have had a CT scan, plus several mammograms and several X-rays over a period of 10 years and do a lot of business airplane travel. It is obvious that those people have a much higher risk of cancer than those who avoid all types of radiation.

ABC news reported that Dr. Len Lichtenfeld, deputy chief medical officer of the American Cancer Society, said that radiation from these scans is not inconsequential and can cause cancer later in life. Why then doesn't the medical system explain to all patients the dangers of mammograms? Why do we see every day more mammography centers opening in every community and more mammo buses going from corporation to corporation offering convenient mammogram tests directly outside their offices? In my opinion, the reason is simple, MONEY! There is so much money to be made in cancer screening and treatment that it is obvious these cancer clinics offer such convenient services. Most businesses provide this as a free benefit to their employees without knowing the harm this "benefit" causes to their employees.

Mammograms have another serious problem that patients don't know. There is a very high number of false positives and false negatives. For this reason many doctors are wondering ... Is mammography an effective tool to detect breast cancer? Some critics say no, and a study of 60,000 women in Switzerland showed that 70% of tumors detected by mammography were actually not tumors according to the biopsies done to these people. This is part of the category of false positives. Worst of all is that this leads to many unnecessary biopsies and procedures. It also creates unnecessary stress on the patient when the oncologist says that the mammography detected a shadow that has to be reviewed in more detail. One good thing about these false positives is the money it brings to the clinics because biopsies are not cheap and someone has to pay for them. If you have insurance, you are still paying for it one way or another. One way is by the ever rising cost of health insurance year after year.

At the same time, the book "The Politics of Cancer" by Dr. Samuel S. Epstein speaks of false negatives. In this book Dr. Epstein explains that in women 40 to 49 years, one in four instances of cancer is not detected by mammography. The National Cancer Institute puts the false negative rates even higher than 40% among this age group. The researchers found that the breast tissue of young women is denser, making it difficult to detect tumors. That is why false negatives occur more often in pre-menopausal women.

The dangers of radiation from such medical devices have been documented by the FDA, NCI and countless scientific studies. In 1976 for example, mammography equipment produced between 5 and 10 RADs (or Radiation Absorbed Dosis) for each projection. The new machines emanate only one RAD but this radiation exposure increases the risk of breast cancer by 1% according to Dr. Frank Rauscher who was the deputy director of the NCI.

Dr. Russell Blaylock, MD, estimates that each annual mammogram increases the risk of breast cancer by 2%. This corresponds to a 20% risk in a period of 10 years. In the 60's and 70's this risk was never explained to patients including those high risk women who were having 10 mammograms per year. Dr. Blaylock says the little benefit that mammography provides does not justify the long-term risk.

Dr. John W Gofman who is an authority on the effects of ionizing radiation, estimated that 75% of cases of breast cancer can be prevented if exposure to ionizing radiation is limited. This includes mammograms, X-rays, CT scans and other medical and dental sources.

According to statistics, since mammography was instituted as the norm for breast cancer screening the incident of breast cancer called Ductal Carcinoma in Situ (DCIS) has increased by over 300% and it is believed that approximately 200% of this increase is due to mammography. Above all, during mammogram screening, the breasts are almost flattened from top to bottom and side to side. This may over stimulate existing cancer cells and cause metastases. This means that if a patient goes for a normal breast examination and does not know that she already has a small tumor, this over stimulation can multiply that small tumor and spread more rapidly throughout the breast area. That means good business for them and bad news for you. But who cares about you, right?

A Canadian national study of breast cancer in 1992 showed that mammography had no positive effect on mortality in women between 40 and 50 years old. Moreover, this study suggested that women in this age group are more likely to die from mammograms.

I assume you are wondering, ok then, what can I do to detect breast cancer? There is a technology called Thermography, which is FDA approved. This is a procedure that uses a thermal camera that takes one or more images of the breast area from 3-5 feet away. These images are examined by a doctor or medical expert with the help of a computer. This procedure does not use X-rays or any harmful radiation and has no side effects. The only bad thing about Thermography is that not all health insurance companies cover this procedure and therefore the patient has to cover the cost from her own pocket. But don't be discouraged because some insurance companies do cover them. If your health insurance does not cover it I suggest you make an effort to get the money and pay out of pocket. The risk of mammograms is too high and it is preferable to pay US$130 to US$170 than to have to risk developing breast cancer due to the cumulative effect of multiple mammograms over the years. Educate yourself on this subject and don't let a cancer clinic or mammography center convince you to endure a mammogram with its high percentage of false positives and the possibility of causing metastasis on an existing tumor. Remember that it is your decision and not the doctor's. You have every right to reject conventional barbaric methods of cancer treatment, not only mammograms but also chemotherapy and radiation. Educating yourself goes a long way and will help you have a more professional conversation with your doctor. A doctor is always going to try to convince you to have a mammogram under the promise that they are safe and effective, but if you ask the right questions and put the doctor or the nurse on the spot, the conversation may be a little different. Don't be intimidated if your doctor says something like *"Where did you read that information? The internet? Don't believe everything you read in the internet"* with a sentence similar to this most doctors will convince you to get the test done. So, before your doctor says that to you, educate yourself and bring literature from medical journals and scientific studies and show him/her the risks as explained by the experts in the radiology field. It is your life so make sure you have all the facts in front of you. Don't trust 100% of your health to the medical system because deaths from medical errors persist as the #3 killer in the US, claiming the lives of more than 400,000 people each year.

At a senate hearing in July 2014, members explained the devastating loss of human life (more than 1,000 people each day) as well as the cost to the tax payers which is close to $1 trillion dollars each year. The problem doesn't stop there because for each 1,000 people that die each day, there are also about 10,000 serious complications cases reported each day that are caused by medical errors which in many cases result in permanent brain damage or paralysis among others. I don't want to scare you but I do want to make you aware that medical errors are a huge problem and knowing about them will make you a more informed patient for you and your children. By the way, most States have a law suit cap for medical errors so don't dream if you think you can sue a doctor or a pharmaceutical company for millions of dollars because the law is not on your side when it comes to compensation. The law favors the corporations more than it favors you. Thank the law makers for this.

Here is an example of medical errors in the radiation field. In 2009, more than 200 stroke patients at Cedars-Sinai Medical Center, in Los Angeles, began suffering from hair loss and skin redness after getting head CT scans. An FDA investigation found that technicians exposed these patients with eight times the appropriate dose of radiation level. This is equivalent to about 50,000 X-rays and according to the US Nuclear Regulatory Commission this dose can kill a person if the radiation exposure is done to the entire body.

Another example of medical errors in this field is the case of Jacoby Roth, a 2 year old boy who was taken to the emergency room in 2008 when he fell off his bed and hit his head. The emergency room technician performed multiple CT scans. This caused a massive radiation overdose potentially harming him for the rest of his life. There is clear evidence that children are at higher risk because their small bodies are more sensitive to radiation than adults. The biggest problem is that children are exposed to adult doses of radiation instead of pediatric doses. These machines have level controls but sometimes technicians forget to adjust the level for the proper patient. Some doctors are taking note and waking up to the dangers of CT scans but there is a money issue here; for every CT scan performed, the hospital makes a good chunk of money which helps them pay for their multi-million dollar equipment. Remember that you have to take control of your health by educating yourself. I recommend you to read other books on this subject along with articles from independent studies and clinical studies that are non-biased on this subject so you can make an informed decision rather than just doing what the doctor says. Remember that doctors don't know everything and…. What your doctor doesn't know, may be killing you.

pH - Potential Hydrogen

This chapter is probably the most important for people suffering from cancer or those with a history of cancer in the family. It is obviously also important for everyone else, like people suffering from osteoporosis, arthritis and obesity. On this particular subject you will find many books on the health books market. One of these books is "Alkalize or Die" by Dr. Theodore Baroody. In this book Dr. Baroody explains that almost all diseases and ailments are caused by an acid system with high deficiency in alkaline parts needed to balance the pH levels. The human body must have a pH near 7.0. Back in high school we learned that the pH levels range from 1 to 14. We also learned that a pH of 1 is so powerful that it can make a hole on an iron bar and a pH of 14 is highly alkaline. The ideal pH of the human body is 7.36. When the blood pH is maintained between 7 and 7.4 you don't have to worry about getting cancer or any other chronic disease because disease cannot live in an alkaline rich environment. When the body is in this range, all the organs, the immune system, cells and molecules work in harmony and balance. As the body becomes more acidic, a number of problems including body weight, acne, aches and pain in different parts of the body are reflected as inflammation, loss of calcium in bones and many other problems. The acid is formed for several reasons including the environment, stress and others but the most common and easy way comes from the food we eat daily. Acid foods create an imbalance in the pH and if the person continues to eat acid foods, the body will ultimately go into acidosis which is an excessively acid condition of the body fluids and tissues. When this happens the body goes into survival mode and gets calcium from the largest source in the body, the bones. And guess what happens when your bones are robbed from the calcium it needs? That's right....Osteoporosis. But that's not the only problem you need to worry about. If your blood pH is too acidic, your body becomes a feeding ground for cancer cells. This is why you need to know the foods you are eating and make an effort to change your habits before it's too late.

The most acidic foods are those found in processed foods with lots of preservatives, dyes, sugar and artificial flavors. Remember that almost 80% of the foods sold in supermarkets today are highly processed and can last months and even years on the shelves. People call a can of soup "food"; I call it "potential poison". If a product can last years on the shelves do you really believe that product is good for you? Do you know how hard the digestive system and the liver have to work to digest and filter that food? In many cases, that food cannot be filtered and absorbed so the liver traps it in the form of fat. Processed foods are the worst kind but products with high sugar content and refined carbohydrates are just as bad because those products are converted to glucose very quickly. Just remember this….. Sugar turns into acid ash inside your body. You can imagine what happens when you eat too much sugar or refined carbohydrates; if you said cancer, you guessed correctly.

The good news is that the pH can be raised and balanced relatively easy. The steps are simple for some and more difficult for others. It all depends on you but you need to understand that cancer, obesity and heart disease cannot be cured or reversed without making drastic changes to your diet. You need to change your eating habits and incorporate a highly alkaline diet or at least a diet that contains 80% alkaline foods and 20% acid foods. This subject is so important that your life depends on it. Cancer is a fungus and it can be removed from your body if you make the changes described in this book and especially the information provided in this chapter. Cancer cells starve in an alkaline rich environment and flourish in an acidic body. This is why you need to embrace this concept and begin to change your life forever. Don't be fool by all the marketing campaign from the food industry.

Alkaline foods

Alkalizing Foods
- Alfalfa - Barley grass - Beet greens - Beets - Carrots - Celery
- Broccoli - Cauliflower - Cabage - Chard greens - Cucumber
- Chlorella - Dandelions - Eggplant - Garlic - Green beens - Kale
- Green peas - Lettuce - Mushrooms - Mustard greens - Onions
- Parsnips - Peas - Peppers - Pumpkin - Radishes - Sea veggies
- Spinach - Green spirulina - Sprouts - Tomatoes - Watercress
- Sweet potatoes - Wheat grass - Wild greens - Kombu - Nori
- Daikon - Maitake - Wakame - Reishi - Shitake - Umeboshi
- Kelp - Mango - Cayene - Papaya - Parsley - Seaweeds - Kiwi
- Asparagus - Passionfruit - Avocado - Bell peppers
- Apple - Apricot - Avocado - Banana (high glycemic)
- Blackberries - Cantaloupe - Cherries - Coconut - Dates - Figs
- Grapes - Grapefruit - Honeydew melon - Lemon - Lime - Pear
- Nectarine - Orange - Peach - Pineapple - Raisins - Raspberries
- Strawberries - Tangerine - Watermelon - Tropical fruits
- Almonds - Chestnuts - Millet - Tempeh - Tofu (fermented)
- Stevia - Chili pepper - Cinnamon - Curry - Ginger - Miso - Herbs
- Sea salt - Tamari - Alkalized water - Apple cider vinegar
- Bee pollen - Green juices - Mineral water - Molasses
- Probiotic cultures - Veggie juices - Fresh made juices
- Calcium (pH 12) - Potassium (pH 14) - Sodium (pH 14)
- Magnesium (pH 9) - Cesium (pH 14)
- Baking soda - Lentils - Citrus juices - Olives - Arugula - Cashews

Acidic foods

Acidic Foods
- White flour (bleached white flour)
- White rice, salt, white sugar
- Cereals with artificial sugars and flavors
- White refined pasta
- Prescription and over the counter medications
- Beer (pH 2.5) - Hard liquor - Wine - Cigarettes
- Meats (beef, pork, chicken)
- Bacon - Lamb - Rabbit - Turkey - Veal - Venison
- Lobster - Clams - Haddok - Mussels - Oyster - Shrimp
- Salmon - Sardines - Sausage -Scallops - Tuna - Cod
- Processed meats - Eggs - Cows milk cheese
- Microwavable foods - Vinegar - Yeast
- Pasteurazied and homogenized milk
- Coffee (pH 4.0) - Cafeinated drinks - Sodas (pH 2.0)
- Peanuts - Pecans - Walnuts - Tahini
- Milk chocolate
- Mermelade - Jelly - Honey
- Mustard - Ketchup - Mayonaise - Butter
- Green plaintains
- Blueberries - Rasberries - Cranberries
- Currants - Canned or glazed fruits
- Corn - Soda crackers - Cornstarch - Macaroni
- Wheat germ - Rye - Rice cakes - Quinoa - Kamut

Cancer Summary

- Eliminate or reduce sugar consumption. Sugar feeds cancer cells, that's a scientific fact.
- Drink lots of water, lemon, grapefruit and fresh squeezed lemonade (These raise the pH level in your blood and therefore alkalizes your body)
- Reduce or eliminate consumption of red meat and other fatty meats
- Do not eat processed meats (pepperoni, sausage, salami, sausage, bacon, ham). These contain sodium nitrates and nitrites which have been shown to increase the risk of pancreatic cancer by 67% and double the risk of colorectal cancer.
- Children have a 300% increase risk of brain tumors when eating hot dogs with sodium nitrates and nitrites.
- Grilling introduces a potent carcinogenic called Heterocyclic Amine. Pre-cook before grilling for a safer alternative.
- Acrylamides are cancer causing chemicals that are also formed when foods are grilled, fried or roasted at high temp.
- Reduce stress (very important)
- Eliminate High Fructose Corn Syrup from your diet
- Don't use too much makeup or better yet, change your makeup with natural products. The FDA doesn't control cosmetic products and there are many ingredients that are banned from the food supply but they are still allowed in cosmetic products.
- Do not eat anything with trans fats or hydrogenated fats
- Increase fiber, fruits and vegetables in your daily diet
- Eliminate cow's milk from your diet. It is highly acidic. Drink Almond or rice milk instead
- Drink smoothies made by yourself (use organic fruits if possible and add vegetables, flax seed and chia seeds)
- Take vitamin C, D3 and K

- Vitamin C in high doses has shown to fight cancer cells. Read about Dr Linus Polin who recommended very high doses of this vitamin to his patients (30,000mg and higher)

- Eat high alkaline foods and reduce foods that are converted to acid ash in your body

- Eliminate the consumption of artificial sugars, artificial colors and flavors

- Avoid bromated flour in the form of Potassium Bromate. This is used in flour to make it bulk up and rise up more quickly and decreases baking time. This ingredient is a carcinogenic banned in Europe, Canada and even China. US law doesn't require it to be listed as a separate ingredient. Thanks to corrupt politicians.

- Detox your body, especially the liver and the colon

- Eat broccoli, cauliflower, cabbage, Bok Choy, Cabbage, Spinach, Romaine lettuce and other green vegetables.

- Eat legumes such as lentils, peas and organic soy.

- Eat Flaxseed, Garlic, Onion, Grapes, Tomatoes, Green Tea, Blueberries, Strawberries, Blackberries.

- Eat sour apple juice made with water, not milk.

- Take a green super food mix. If you're new to this just mix the powder with 70% water and 30% orange juice or apple juice. This elevates the pH level. I buy a berry flavor called Amazing Grass green super food. Drink a cup or two every day.

- Drink 12-16 ounces of water with lemon (no sugar) upon rising every single day. Drink this water with every meal. DO NOT drink any sodas, not even the diet ones, they are worse.

- Practice yoga, Tai Chi, Qi Qong and others who help reduce stress. Stress kills and causes disease.

- Avoid watching bad news or videos that cause emotional stress. Remember, stress causes your body to get acidic

- Laugh. Try watching funny movies that make you laugh hard. There have been several studies on the benefits of laughter and reduction of cancerous tumors. Laugh releases endorphins that kill cancer cells.

- Try to have a clear mind with positive thoughts. The book "The Secret" talks about this. It works.

ALZHEIMER'S

This disease is the most common form of dementia in older adults accounting for 60% to 80% of all cases. Dementia is basically a loss of brain function which typically develops during the golden years. It is a broad term for neurological conditions that involve some type of serious mental impairment such as memory loss, confusion or personality changes. This disease didn't make the top 10 causes of death in the Unites States until the early 1990's. Today it is the number 6 cause of death in the United States and other industrialized nations. This disease kills approximately 85,000 Americans each year according to the death statistics published by the CDC in 2013. It is believed that this disease will almost quadruple in the next 50 years. When this occurs, nearly 1 in every 45 Americans will be afflicted with this disease. Some experts believe that Alzheimer's may be a form of type 3 diabetes due to its connection to brain insulin resistance and its corresponding inflammation. This was published in the Journal of Alzheimer's Disease. This insulin resistance prevents some lipids or fats from properly getting metabolized and over time this causes stress and inflammation which in turn cause the symptoms commonly known as dementia. So, if Alzheimer's is similar to diabetes, it shouldn't surprise us that these diseases became prevalent or significant in the early 1990's because sugar in the form of High Fructose Corn Syrup was introduced in the mass production of processed foods in the 1980's. As I mentioned before, HFCS is a man made sugar that has been linked to many diseases.

The chances of developing Alzheimer's doubles every five years from age 65 to 85. If you don't make changes to your diet, sleep better and start exercising your mind with brain games and activities to keep you busy and alert, your mind will eventually falter and slowly get worse as each year passes. Don't settle for this, your life is worth living it to its fullest. You owe it to your family, your grand kids and to yourself.

Symptoms

Okay so let's talk about symptoms. The first signs of this disease may be mild confusion and occasional forgetfulness. However, overtime, this progresses into constant memory loss especially recent memories. Now, remember that every person is different and the symptoms and the rate at which they occur varies from person to person. If you have Alzheimer's you or your spouse may notice that you are having a difficult time remembering things and organizing your thoughts. Memory is the first thing that you may notice but you may not notice changes in your mood; this will be something your spouse or loved ones will notice and be affected once it grows into brain malfunction, disorientation and mental confusion. Now, everyone has occasional minor memory issues such as forgetting where you put your keys or eye glasses or even forgetting a name of person you haven't seeing for a while. What's not normal is the repeating of statements and questions over and over during a normal conversation. Or forgetting appointments and conversations that occurred just a day or two ago or even forgetting the names of your family members. Other symptoms are related to the inability to clearly speak and write. Normal thinking and reasoning is also affected as well as making judgment calls and everyday decisions. Performing familiar tasks such as cooking a meal or even bathing are more extreme but unfortunately common in seniors at much earlier ages than ever before. This is very alarming but no one in the medical establishment seems to be connecting the dots and raising a red flag. Just to be clear, I'm not talking about the doctors; I'm talking about the medical system which in my opinion, is heavily influenced and manipulated by the pharmaceutical industry which only cares about patching the problem instead of focusing on the real cure. There are a few FDA approved drugs available for Alzheimer's patients but according to independent studies and Placebo tests, they do nothing to mitigate this deadly disease, but it does great damage to the liver and other organs due to the side effects of these drugs. I am predicting based on my research and reading many articles and scientific journals, that if nothing changes in the food supply and life continues the way it is today, in the next 10-15 years there will be a health crisis of great magnitude and people in their 40's will need the medical attention and medicines that people in their 70's and 80's are taking today.

Doctor Russell Blaylock said something similar a few years ago. This is not rocket science folks. When you change real and fresh food with highly processed packaged food, common sense should tell you that nothing good comes out from this change. Some people tell me that I'm extreme because I don't let my kids eat at McDonalds or drink soda; well I believe letting your kids eat and drink these so called "foods" is a lot more extreme, especially once you understand the damage these "foods" can cause after long term consumption. Now, if you want to enjoy a soda once or twice a year, that's ok, it won't kill you. But if you allow your children to drink a soda every other day or even once a week, you better start saving for their future medical bills related to obesity, diabetes, Alzheimer's and other degenerative diseases. Don't tell me I didn't warn you.

Prevention

Prevention should be your number one priority for this and other degenerative diseases. There are several things you can do to prevent this disease and stay away from any of the pharmaceutical drugs that are currently offered. One of the most important ones is regular exercise. This alone will help you clear your mind, move all the cells in your body and maintain a healthy heart which is your main engine. When you walk or jog regularly, all the cells in your body are activated and vitamins and minerals from your food get properly distributed and transported throughout your body. Staying active is the single most important thing you should do to keep your mind alert and fresh. When you walk, try to do it briskly and moving your hands up and down like a Russian marching soldier. This will help the lymphatic system move all the toxins and waste from the blood stream into your body's elimination channels.

Taking vitamin D3 has been shown to lower the risk of many chronic diseases including heart disease, cancer, diabetes, stroke and Alzheimer's. A study by the Angers University Hospital in France demonstrated the importance of vitamin D for the cognitive health of women as they age. They provided evidence that vitamin D intake is associated with lower risk of developing Alzheimer's disease. As I mentioned before, most Americans are deficient in vitamin D; no wonder why the United States is the country with the highest level of this disease.

Green tea and red wine can also help in the prevention of this disease. According to an article in naturalnews.com, bioactive compounds found in green tea and red wine halt Alzheimer's disease progression. Researchers from the University of Leeds in the UK found that the natural chemicals found in green tea and red wine help prevent this deadly disease because these chemicals disrupt the accumulation of Amyloid plaque which block the transmission of electrical and chemical transmitters that allow the brain to store information, maintain cognitive function and retain memories. Amyloid proteins in the brain form a cluster of toxic and sticky lumps of different shapes. These amyloid clusters or balls latch onto the surface of nerve cells and eventually causes them to malfunction and die.

Obesity also accelerates cognitive decline and memory breakdown. When you are overweight your blood glucose and blood pressure go up causing a rapid decline in cognitive skills like thinking properly and memory. A study on 6,400 participants by the French research institute INSERM confirmed this when they demonstrated that small increase in biomarkers such as blood glucose and blood pressure result in dramatically increased risk of dementia and Alzheimer's. As you can see being obese or even overweight increases your chances of developing many different types of diseases. You need to realize that carrying a belly that makes you look like you are 7 months pregnant is not healthy and you must make changes to your life style before it's too late to reverse a deadly disease. You can't ignore the fact that the mirror is not lying to you. The mirror doesn't have a magnifying effect. So, next time you look in the mirror take a very good look at yourself and decide if you want to live with those extra pounds for the rest of your life and eventually suffer from the diseases mentioned in this book or change your fate and live to be 100 without medicines so you can enjoy your grand kids and great grand kids. The older you get the more difficult it will be to remove those extra pounds and the more prone to diseases you will be. Make an effort to lose weight NOW; you owe it to yourself and your love ones.

Alzheimer's Summary

- This is the # 6 cause of death in the US with an Approximate amount of 85,000 deaths each year
- More than half of the rooms in the nursing homes today are occupied by patients with Alzheimer's. This is pretty sad
- Between 2000 and 2006 the number of deaths from Alzheimer's increased by 47% (According to the CDC). Why isn't anybody talking about this?
- Did you know that the flu shot contains Mercury which is a poison that causes Alzheimer's? The majority of senior citizens get the flu shot every year. Is there a link here? I think so.
- Mercury toxicity symptoms are similar to those of Alzheimer's. Read the letter they make you sign before injecting you with the flu shot poison. Mercury is hidden under the name Thimerosal.
- Approximately 5.3 million Americans have Alzheimer's. It is predicted that this number will triple in 40 years
- *Opinion: Alzheimer's can be prevented and in some cases it can be reversed if extreme detoxification measures are taken.*

How to Prevent Alzheimer's

*This statement has not been evaluated by the FDA

- Avoid or drastically reduce the consumption of MSG

- Avoid eating aspartame and other artificial sweeteners

- Cook in stainless steel pots instead of aluminum

- Do not cook in aluminum pots such as pressure cookers

- Change your dental metal fillings with white amalgam fillings

- Do not eat fish with high mercury content. See appendix for a list of fish with high, medium and low mercury content

- Avoid living near factories that pollute the environment

- Do not get the flu vaccine - Contains mercury in the form of Thimerasol and aluminum

- If you are over 65 years of age, exercise the mind and brain with brain games, Sudoku, cross words and others

- Detoxify your body from mercury and aluminum

- Take vitamin C in large quantities (20,000 mg per day). Take the non-acidic form of vitamin C for better absorption. Read the chapter on vitamin C.

- Stay away from pesticides and household chemicals

OBESITY

This is a disease that affects millions of people in the United States and other industrialized countries. According to the Center for Disease Control and the Journal of the American Medicinal Association (JAMA), approximately one third or 35 percent of adults and 17 percent of children in the United States are obese. Please note that I'm not talking about overweight which affects two thirds of the American public. I'm talking about those who have a body mass index or BMI greater than 30%. If your BMI is 25%-29% you are considered overweight. The table below shows the different BMI percentages based on the height and weight of the person. Find your BMI number on the top and see where you fall. If you are in the obese range, you have to start making changes to your diet and life style. If you don't make any changes, please start saving money for your future medical bills and medicines that you will need to include in your monthly budgetary expenses. That is a fact, not a prediction. As I mentioned before, obesity related diseases include type 2 diabetes, heart disease, stroke, certain types of cancer and eventually Alzheimer's. It is estimated that the annual medical cost of obesity in the United States is $148 billion US dollars.

BMI	19	20	21	22	23	24	25	26	27	28	29	30	31	32	33	34	35
Height	Weight In Pounds															
4'10"	91	96	100	105	110	115	119	124	129	134	138	143	148	153	158	162	167
4'11"	94	99	104	109	114	119	124	128	133	138	143	148	153	158	163	168	173
5'	97	102	107	112	118	123	128	133	138	143	148	153	158	163	168	174	179
5'1"	100	106	111	116	122	127	132	137	143	148	153	158	164	169	174	180	185
5'2"	104	109	115	120	126	131	136	142	147	153	158	164	169	175	180	186	191
5'3"	107	113	118	124	130	135	141	146	152	158	163	169	175	180	186	191	197
5'4"	110	116	122	128	134	140	145	151	157	163	169	174	180	186	192	197	204
5'5"	114	120	126	132	138	144	150	156	162	168	174	180	186	192	198	204	210
5'6"	118	124	130	136	142	148	155	161	167	173	179	186	192	198	204	210	216
5'7"	121	127	134	140	146	153	159	166	171	178	185	191	198	204	211	217	223
5'8"	125	131	138	144	151	158	164	171	177	184	190	197	203	210	216	223	230
5'9"	128	135	142	149	155	162	169	176	182	189	196	203	209	216	223	230	236
5'10"	132	139	146	153	160	167	174	181	188	195	202	209	216	222	229	236	243
5'11"	136	143	150	157	165	172	179	186	193	200	208	215	222	229	236	243	250
6'	140	147	154	162	169	177	184	191	199	206	213	221	228	235	242	250	258
6'1"	144	151	159	166	174	182	189	197	204	212	219	227	235	242	250	257	265
6'2"	148	155	163	171	179	186	194	202	210	218	225	233	241	249	256	264	272
6'3"	152	160	168	176	184	192	200	208	216	224	232	240	248	256	264	272	279
	Healthy Weight						Overweight					Obese					

BMI Table for adults

Obesity rates affect some groups more than others according to JAMA.

Non-Hispanic blacks have the highest rates of obesity (47.8%) followed by Hispanics (42.5%), non-Hispanic whites (32.6%) and non-Hispanic Asians (10.8%). Obesity is also different depending on the socioeconomic status. Among non-Hispanic black and Mexican-American men, those with higher incomes have a higher tendency of obesity than those with low income. However, the opposite is true for women. Higher income women are less likely to be obese than low income women. No one knows why but women with college degrees are less likely to be obese than those with less education. One reason could be that more educated women can afford healthier grocery choices and gym memberships. Less educated women are also more likely to have two or more jobs and therefore have less time to cook healthy meals and they find themselves eating out at fast food restaurants more often than they would like to. They also don't have the time to engage in physical exercise. This is sad because these people won't have the money to deal with the health care cost that they will have to endure during their golden years. This also causes a heavy burden on the overall US economy since a great deal of money is spent on health care related to obesity. In fact, in the US along the annual hospital costs for children and young adults related to overweight and obesity has tripled in the past two decades.

So, let's find out why and when the obesity problem started. According to the Center for Disease Control or CDC, between 1980 and 2000, obesity rates doubled among adults, double among children and tripled among adolescents. This is having a huge impact in the US health statistics. So much so that not long ago, type 2 diabetes was believed to affect only adults. Not anymore; In fact, there are some communities where almost half of the pediatric patients are diagnosed with type 2 diabetes. Not too long ago, this rate was close to zero. About Sixty percent of the children considered overweight, ages 5-10, already have at least one risk factor for heart disease. As I explained in the diabetes section of this book, type 2 diabetes increases serious complications in adults such as kidney disease, blindness and amputations. Imagine then how early it will occur on our children. This is a big issue and must be addressed right away but for some reason the media and the medical establishment are more focused on telling us about the recent measles outbreak (which is virtually harmless in most cases) than heavily advertising the fact that our children are getting fatter and sicker each year. They should be trying to find the true root cause of this issue so they can work on preventive measures that will ultimately fix the problem once and for all. The government should be subsidizing healthy foods for the majority of the people to be able to afford more fruits and vegetables instead of the heavily processed and junk foods that the majority of people are eating. Most of us know that poor or unhealthy diet and lack of exercise or physical activity causes you and your children to be overweight. Despite this fact, most people don't eat the recommended 5-6 servings of fruits and vegetables each day and more than 50% of adults don't get enough exercise to gain the health benefits that it provides. The worse thing of all this is that one third of children ages 13-18 don't engage in regular physical activity. Some experts believe that this is mainly due to the electronics era that most industrialized nations are now accustomed to. It is true that most children nowadays are hooked to their smart phones, tablets and TV sets. Another reason that adds to the obesity problem is the heavy competition between fast food restaurants and food companies in general. This competition has brought bigger portions at these restaurants and convenience stores like 7-11 where it is easy to find a big Gulp soda (32 ounces) or a super big Gulp of 44 ounces and even a double gulp which comes in a huge 64 ounce tub. The worse thing is that this type of drinks are loaded with sugar, phosphoric acid and cancer causing caramel color and other ingredients. If you drink one of these tubs and then have a glucose test, you will most likely be diagnosed with diabetes or pre-diabetes. Back in 1955, McDonalds introduced soft drinks in a seven ounce cup. As we all know, today it is not uncommon to find a 32 ounce cup in most of the fast food restaurants. This change increased the calorie count to 300 and added more than 80 grams of sugar. Some of the health advocate groups have joked about holding companies like Coca-Cola and PepsiCo responsible for selling glucose altering drinks because even the 12 ounce cans of soda have enough sugar to spike your blood glucose and cause your pancreas to excrete more insulin than normal to balance the sugar load.

According to a few experts, the replacement of real sugar with High Fructose Corn Syrup or HFCS back in the mid 1980's could be the reason to the increase number of obesity, diabetes and cancer cases in the past 3 decades. As I explained before, HFCS is a form of sugar made from GMO corn which affects many organs of the body including the liver and the pancreas. I am a very analytical person who knows that true statistics don't lie and according to the latest statistics, diabetes, obesity and cancer cases started to grow in the mid to upper 1980's. This correlates with the massive introduction of HFCS and other heavily processed and packaged "foods". It is also the time when bigger portions were introduced. So, in my opinion, you don't need to be a rocket scientist to connect the dots and draw the conclusion that the mentioned "foods" and sugary drinks are the main culprits in obesity rates. If nothing changes, the US population will most likely be 50% obese in the next 10-15 years and its citizens will resemble the characters in the movie, WALL-E, where most of the people are so obese that they have to ride on electric wheel chairs equipped with a tablet that helps them watch TV, play games and order everything they want without having to stand up. They literally have to roll over their comfy chair and crawl if they have to do something else. But wait, some people are already getting to this point, aren't they? In fact, you can find some of those people when you go to the supermarket or mass retail store where they have free electric wheel chairs for the obese. I feel sorry for them because they really don't have a clue what made them so obese to begin with. They are being told that the reason they are obese is because they don't exercise (which is true) and that they are eating too much (which is also true); but they are not being told that the foods they are eating are heavily processed, loaded with artificial sugars, colors and flavor enhancers to make the food taste better. These foods are also full of addictive ingredients that make you want to eat more and more. They also don't know that these "foods" are most likely causing them to gain weight and get sick. All they know is that processed "foods" and "food" from fast food restaurants is very affordable so that's what they normally eat and feed their children. The food companies as well as the pharmaceutical companies have excellent marketing people who do a great job of advertising and promoting their products with fancy labels and colorful packaging. They make the food look beautiful and colorful. But, did you know that many of the products that you see on the shelves and frozen sections have been altered by adding artificial colors? For instance, next time you go to the supermarket, check the label on that amazingly bright farmed salmon or steak displayed on the frozen section. Don't be surprised when you see a label that reads something like "color added" or anything similar. The flesh of wild salmon is pink but the flesh of farmed raised salmon is grey so color is added to make it look as good as wild salmon. Food companies do this because they know that if they display fish and meats the same way they come from the animal, no one will buy them.

So be aware of the deceiving marketing ads and fancy looking packaging. Read the labels and educate yourself about the foods you are eating or feeding your children. At least do it for them because they don't know any better and you are responsible for the food you put on the table.

A good example of reading labels can be found on most of the non-organic infant formula drinks. If you look on the back of the label you will see the ingredients list (which nobody reads). In this list you will be shocked to find out that most of these baby drinks have more than 50% sugar content in the form of corn solids, sucrose and other sugar names. Some of them have artificial sugars which are worse because of the neurotoxic effect I explained in earlier chapters. When it comes to caring for your babies, you have to be particularly careful with the food you feed them because their digestive tract, liver and other organs are in the early development stage of their lives. If they eat too much processed foods and drink sugary drinks, they will fall under the overweight and obese statistics and eventually develop diseases like diabetes, cancer and heart disease. I know it is hard to switch from the great tasting sugary and processed foods but if you don't do it early enough in your life, you will regret it later in life when perhaps it is too late to reverse these deadly diseases.

So how do we reverse obesity? The answer is actually very simple unless you have a medical condition that needs to be treated by a medical doctor. One tip I want to give you is don't engage in any diet that promises to help you lose 10 or 20 pounds in one or two weeks. In my opinion, they are lying to you and their claims are not worth the paper they are printed on. Currently in the United States, one third of all women and one fourth of all men are doing some type of diet. But this is not new, men and women have been dieting for decades without success. People place a lot of hope in these diet programs because it appeals to them and they truly believe they are going to lose weight. Unfortunately, according to the statistics, most of the people who go on a diet and lose weight end up gaining more weight than when they started the diet. For this reason I don't believe in any diet even if they guarantee results that are too good to be true. The best way to lose weight and keep it off is by eating smaller portions a few times a day. My recommendation is to drink 12-16 ounces of water upon rising. This alone will do wonders. Eat a decent size breakfast with lots of protein and fruits and another 12-16 ounces of look warm water, followed by a snack around 10am (fruits, nuts or a smoothie). Lunch should be somewhat proportional to your body size but don't eat more than a plate full. If you go to a lunch buffet, make sure it only occurs once a year or twice at the most, because those places make you eat a lot more than normal as you may already know. Eat another snack around 4pm and finally, eat a light dinner with vegetables and fruits. Don't forget to drink water at every meal and snack time and do not eat three hours before bedtime. The worst thing you can do is eating a large meal at dinner time and a small breakfast. This will trigger a response similar to hibernation while you sleep because the body will remember that your breakfast will be very small and lacking the protein it needs and will automatically store most of your dinner meal as fat while you sleep. So, eating a small breakfast is something you need to avoid doing long term. Another thing that you must do if you want to lose weight is to be active. Sitting on your couch during or after your dinner is not going to help you lose weight so get up and get moving. You can start walking and little by little increase your pace until you start jogging. The key is to sweat those extra pounds by doing some type of exercise. Remember one thing – every calorie you eat has to be burn, period. If you consume 3,000 calories per day, you will never lose weight if you don't burn more than those 3,000 calories per day. Trust me, 3,000 calories are very easy to ingest but they take a lot of effort to burn. The more fat cells you have the harder it is to burn calories and the slower your metabolism will be. You need to take a good look at your calorie intake and try your best to take less than what you are burning. Now, not all calories are the same. For instance, 90 calories from a medium apple is not the same as 90 calories from a bite of a sneaker bar. In the next few pages you will find a summary of these and other tips that will help you lose weight and avoid most of the degenerative diseases that are caused by being overweight. Don't get discourage if you're not losing weight as quickly as you would like to. Remember, it is not realistic to think that you can lose weight by continuing to eat the way you are eating now and without engaging in any physical activity. Diets don't work long term. In the next few pages you will find exercise routines that have been especially designed by my good friend and excellent Personal Trainer, Fabian Valencia. These exercise programs are designed for those who want to lose weight at home or at the gym. As always, please check with your medical doctor to make sure these exercises are right for you.

Obesity summary

- 60 million adults in the United States are obese
- 9 million children ages 6 to 17 are overweight
- 8 in 10 Americans 25 and older are overweight
- 80% of diabetes cases are associated with obesity
- 70% of cardiovascular diseases are related to obesity
- 42% of people with breast and colon cancer are obese
- 33% of black and Hispanic children are obese
- Studies indicate that 1 in 4 children are overweight and have signs of type 2 diabetes
- Of the children diagnosed with type 2 diabetes, 85% are obese. Get your kids moving every day.

How to lose weight*

*This statement has not been evaluated by the FDA

- Follow the exercise routines designed by Fabian Valencia, BSES and personal trainer, see next section for details
- Drink 1 to 2 glasses of water upon rising (add a few drops of lemon to raise the alkalinity level). Don't add sugar please.
- Eat a big breakfast with protein. Avoid eating too many carbohydrates
- Do a colon and liver cleanse by juicing for 3-5 days. See section on juicing
- Do not eat 3 hours before bedtime

- Measure the amount of calories you eat daily and make sure you burn calories by walking or running. If your consumption of calories succeeds the amount being burned, you will gain weight, period.

- Eat small meals 5-6 times a day. Avoid eating too much animal protein like meats and dairy

- Eat green salads every day or drink green super foods. Your local health food store sells different kinds in powder form

- Drink 8-10 glasses of filtered water a day. Don't forget to add a few drops of lemon. You can also add slices of cucumber, orange or apple to your sports bottle

- Do not drink sodas of any kind including diet sodas. A chemical called 4-Methylimidazole or 4-MI is formed when making the caramel color used in sodas. This chemical has been shown to cause cancer.

- Never eat at fast food restaurants. You should know this.

- Avoid High Fructose Corn Syrup (HFCS). Read the labels

- No artificial sweeteners unless you want to slowly kill your brain cells

- Walk at least 45 minutes a day. Make sure you sweat

- Avoid or eliminate white flour, especially brominated flour

- Drink at least one glass of green tea a day

- Take digestive enzymes

- Take probiotics daily

- Fast 1 or 2 times per month (water or homemade juice only)

- Eat slowly. Chew 25 to 30 times each spoon full

- Breathe deeply for one minute twice daily. This is very important because it help the lymphatic system to move toxins out of the blood stream. It also helps with stress

- Eat foods high in fiber. Flax seed, Chia seeds, Oat meal, Aloe

- Do not eat anything fried
- Say no to processed foods as much as possible
- Don't follow diets. Exercise instead
- Join a gym and MOVE
- Do a liquid diet for 10 days based on extracted juice, water and smoothies without milk (you can use Greek yogurt)

How to lose Weight

A professional opinion by Fabian Valencia, Acute Leukemia survivor

Over the years I've dedicated part of my professional career in developing exercises and meal plans to help people lose weight. I am often asked to guide people of all ages to help them develop an exercise plan that is both, easy and fast, to achieve results in a short period of time. Most people don't realize how challenging this can be because every person is different and an exercise plan that is designed for one person may not work for another. This is hard for people to understand because they want to lose weight very rapidly without too much effort and that can be dangerous. The human body was designed to move and be active, not to eat large quantities of food and then sit down and wait for the body to digest all that food; sorry it doesn't work that way, unless of course, you want to gain weight and be depressed. Did you know that weight gain causes depression? In this chapter of the book I want to provide you with the tools necessary to lose weight in a healthy more sustainable way. I will provide you with exercise plans that fit most people's life styles. My passion is to help others improve their health and wellness. As always, consult your physician before beginning an exercise program. If you experience any pain or difficulty with these exercises, stop and consult your health provider.

A little bit about me

I am 38 years old, born in Chicago and raised in south Florida. I graduated from the University of Florida with a Bachelor's degree in Exercise Science with a focus on fitness and wellness. I have always had an appreciation for exercise and the benefits that come along with keeping a healthy, active lifestyle. In college, this appreciation turned into true passion as I found myself with this strong desire to motivate people to make better choices about their health and to encourage them to get up and move. I learned through many years of trial and error, that if I could help people move well, eat well, and think well, they would feel well.

Fast -forward several years and out of the blue I began feeling incredibly fatigued, with massive headaches and shortness of breath. I was diagnosed with Acute Leukemia (ALL) and began treatment that Christmas. I suffered through relapses, a bone marrow transplant, graft versus host disease (cGVHD) and many complications from my treatment. The irony was that I was better at telling my clients what to do than following my own advice. My nutrition needed a great deal of improvement. So I started reading more and more about how the food we eat is not simply fuel, but has an enormous impact for optimal long-term health. I currently follow many of the recommendations provided by Mr. Aramburo in this book. I strongly believe that it was my desire to keep exercising (I was the only patient in the hospital who was doing pushups in his room and lunges on my floor and walking the stairs), my support structure (wonderful wife, family and friends), and improvement in my nutrition that have given me another shot at life.

In the next few pages I have prepared a few daily routines that will help you get out of the couch and move to gain the health that you deserve. I hope you follow these recommendations and help me transmit this message of exercise and health with your friends and family so they can also enjoy a life with purpose, health and vitality.

Section 1

Let's Start Moving

It is well understood that exercise is good for your mental and physical health. For the sedentary person, it is very easy to add a little exercise into your daily life. It is not mandatory to workout at a gym for an hour a day, every day. Just a little bit of activity may add up if you do it frequently. So get up and move. Start by walking more. Park your car farther away from your destination. Anywhere there are stairs, use them instead of the elevator. Walk your dog more frequently and longer throughout the day. Vacuum your home more often. Go to your friend's yoga class (dance, pilates, etc...). Try a free week at your local gym (they always mail flyers). Do a walk for charity. Plan more trips to the park with your family and friends. If you ride the bus to work, get off at a stop just before yours and walk the rest of the way. If you have access to a pool and can swim, take a dip. Carry your bags while grocery shopping. Play catch (or any sport) with your kids. If you work in an office, skip the emails and get up and speak with the person in your office. These are just a few suggestions to get you started in finding more ways to put exercise and activity in your life. If you are ready for a more regimented routine, then check out the next section.

Section 2

Density Training for Weight Loss

Ever since I began Personal Training, I have used some form of density training with my clients. When I say density training, I'm talking about the ability to do more work within an allotted time frame. This is also known as work capacity. My clients would pay me by the half hour or hour and they wanted results quickly. Density training along with a healthy diet has always been a great way to improve fitness and lose weight. There are two simple ways to work on density training: you can have a set time and try and do more work (let's call it Method 1) or you can decide how much work you want to accomplish and attempt to do it as quickly as possible (Method 2). Please make sure to warm up with some light exercise such as walking, marching or jogging in place, jumping jacks or rope skips. The warm up you choose should be light and easy to prepare you mentally and physically for the workout.

Method 1: Set your own time

Example A - 10 min time limit

Walking Lunges:

Beginner: 5 steps each leg

Intermediate: 10 steps each

Advanced: 15 steps each

Pushups:

Beginner: 5 regular or 10 on your knees

Intermediate: 10 reps

Advanced: 20 reps

Score = Total steps of walking lunges and pushups

Start your watch (or the timer app on your phone) and do a set of walking lunges and then a set of pushups and go back and forth until you reach ten minutes. Rest as needed and the clock is continuous. If you are new to this type of training or just new to exercise in general, start out with low reps (5 steps each leg and 5 pushups for example). You can use dumbbells with the walking lunges. The weight for the walking lunges should be light, something you could do comfortably for 20 steps. The person who doesn't work out at a gym or prefers not to, would simply use bodyweight for the walking lunges. Once you have a score, you have a benchmark to try and beat. For example, if you complete 30 steps with the lunges and 30 reps with the pushups, your score is 60. The next time you try this workout you will try and beat your score of 60, it's pretty simple. Try this method several times before moving onto method 2 or increasing the time on method 1.

Method 2: Set amount of work

Walking Lunges x 100 steps

Pushups x 50 reps

Time to complete:

For simplicity, we will use the above exercises from method 1. With this method of density training, you designate how much work you want to complete (total reps or distance traveled if you want to add an aerobic exercise like running a quarter mile instead of lunges) and you time it. Rest as needed and break up the work however you want. The goal is to beat your previous time.

7 Day Routine

Monday

Circuit

Walking Lunges: 20 reps (Can be done with weights)

Planks with very light knee tap: 15 reps

Pushups: 10 reps

10 min - Score is total reps

Tuesday

Go for a brisk walk or light jog and walk (jog for a little and then walk to recover) 30 – 60 min

Wednesday

Descending Ladder: Reps Start at 10 each, then 9 each, then 8 and so on down to 1 each

Jumping Jacks, Air Squats, Sit Ups

Thursday

Brisk walk, bike ride, take a dip in the pool

Friday

First minute: 20 seconds of Mountain Climbers, 40 seconds rest

Second minute: 20 seconds of Rope Skips, 40 seconds rest

Third minute: 20 seconds of Boxer Shuffles, 40 seconds rest

Fourth minute: 20 seconds of Get Ups*, 40 seconds rest

Repeat 2 – 3 times

*Get Ups are not really a name, it's what I want you to do. Lie down on the floor (clean and safe area) and stand up. It's that simple. You can lay face up or down or alternate – whatever you want.

**Challenge yourself by slowly increasing the time you spend exercising each minute (Example: 20 seconds first two weeks, then 25 seconds the next two weeks...)

Saturday and Sunday

Go to the park, have fun with your family and friends, stay off the couch. Walk and run with your kids.

Tips for Success

- Warm up with some easy activity dependent on your current activity level (walking outside, pushups, squats, jump rope, jumping jacks). You should not feel exhausted, but ready to workout.
- Get a stopwatch/timer or app for your phone.
- Get a journal or notebook to keep track of your workouts; consistency is key. This will help you measure your progress, make notes on how the workout felt and how you felt before and after the workout (ex. didn't sleep well, just tried to get through or feel really good and killed it, time to change exercises, etc...)
- Start out slow and with simple exercises you feel comfortable with. Find your comfort zone before you start pushing your limits. If possible seek out the aid of a fitness professional (trainer, coach, etc.) to make sure your technique is appropriate for you (not everyone should move exactly the same way because of limb length, previous injuries, joint architecture, etc...)
- Create variety in your training to force adaptation and decrease mental staleness: this can be done by increasing weight, changing the exercises, changing the order of exercises, making the exercises more difficult (knee pushup to regular pushup to incline pushup), adding more time for Method 1, changing the amount of work to be completed in Method 2.
- Change the environment. Do your workout in the park or the beach.
- Train with a friend or family member. Having a training partner will help you stay accountable and may improve your performance.

VACCINES

This is a very touchy and controversial subject and many of the medical doctors who have questioned the effectiveness and benefits of vaccines have been ridiculed and stripped out of their medical license. I feel bad for them because they are actually doing a good deed for the community. In the next few pages I will give you a quick introduction to vaccines along with history and statistics about most of the vaccines. I don't intend to be an expert on this subject but I will provide you with scientific proof and data from doctors, scientists and experts in the field of vaccines. My goal in this chapter is to educate you and provide you with the tools necessary to take it to the next level so you can learn more from the experts and make an educated decision when it comes to vaccines. I will provide you with names of several books written on this subject; some of which were written by certified medical doctors who used to believe on the efficacy of vaccines and today are totally against them. Please note that before you make a decision to change your current belief on this subject, you should consult your primary medical doctor or your children's pediatrician. But don't just listen to what they have to say; educate yourself on this subject and make the best educated decision for the future health of your children and yourself. If vaccines were made with just a few non-toxic ingredients and their side effects weren't so serious, I wouldn't object to them.

The majority of the people don't question anything related to vaccines because we have been indoctrinated to believe that vaccines are the answer to multiple diseases and conditions. This could not be further from the truth. Please watch the following documentaries:

- Bought by Jeff Hays
- The Greater Good movie
- Vaccination: The hidden Truth

In an article from doctor Mercola's website at mercola.com he describes how vaccines are a $30 billion dollar industry. There are basically four companies that rule the world of vaccines; they are: Pfizer, Merck, GlaxoSmithKline and Sanofi Pasteur. Most people assume that vaccines are perfectly safe. If this is true, the government must be 100% sure that vaccines are safe as well, right? Sorry, not so. In 1986 the government established the Vaccine Injury Compensation Program (VICP) which is a program where vaccine injury claims are decided in a federal vaccine court to compensate vaccine victims. For years, this court has settled many cases of brain inflammation and permanent brain damage including symptoms of autism. They have paid millions of dollars to basically keep this issue as low profile as possible and away from the public knowledge. Fortunately for us, there are a few groups working to make sure these vaccine injuries don't go silent and most importantly to educate the public to make informed decisions when it comes to their children's health and well being. One of these groups is the National Vaccine Information Center (NVIC), a non-profit organization that advocates for vaccine safety and informed protection in the public health system. Their website is www.NVIC.org Please help them by donating to their good cause of helping people make informed decisions.

The reason the VICP was established in 1986 is because in that same year the government signed a new law called National Childhood Vaccine Protection Injury Act. The name sounds like this law was signed to protect the well being of the children from any vaccine injury. Sorry, not so. This law actually protects the vaccine manufacturers, pediatricians and any other vaccine provider from almost any lawsuit or liability for injuries and deaths caused by government mandated vaccines. Wow! So do you really think the vaccine manufacturers have enough incentives to make vaccines safe? I don't believe so. Since 1986 they have a free ticket to make whatever they want, safe or not. Think about it folks; if they are not liable for any injuries or deaths, why worry about making them 100% safe? Or even 80% safe. In my opinion, these vaccine manufacturers worry more about the profit that vaccines bring to their bottom line than your child's life. If vaccines are so safe, then why has the government setup a federal compensation program to handle the permanent injuries they cause? Please watch the documentary "Bought" and see the corruption that exists in the government and big Pharma. You will be disgusted and sad.

A great majority of vaccine reactions are not reported to the federal Vaccine

Adverse Event Reporting System (VAERS) because some cases are difficult to connect the reactions to the vaccine due to the time frame in which they occur. For instance, if a reaction is reported within hours of the vaccine and it is reported as dramatic or life threatening and the child is taken to the emergency room, only then the case may be a candidate for the vaccine court. The problem is that most reactions don't occur within hours of the vaccine; they may occur the next day or two or even two weeks later. Those cases are viewed as coincidental and not related to the vaccine. Unfortunately, most parents believe it as such and only connect the dots when it is too late to reverse any side effects from these dangerous drugs and the child is left with lifelong chronic illness, disability and permanent brain damage. CDC's database, VAERS, lists more than 8,000 different adverse vaccine reactions ranging from swelling of the injected area to autism, coma and death. It is believed that the number of vaccine reactions is much higher than this but as I explained earlier, the majority of the cases are deemed as coincidental and never reported to the CDC.

Most pediatricians and other vaccine providers have good intentions and truly believe that vaccines are perfectly safe; perhaps because they never questioned the effectiveness of vaccines or maybe because they just don't have the time to keep current with the real science of vaccines or the time to even understand the public health policy and vaccine policy. This is sad because most parents rely on the doctors to care for their children; but, as someone once said, "What your doctor doesn't know may be killing you" maybe true when it comes to vaccines and other drugs. Medical doctors are practically hindered by the medical system and the insurance companies on all aspects. If they deviate from the current procedures or policies, they face being isolated, ridiculed, criticized and even lose their professional license. They also have to pay high living costs and malpractice insurance, so they have to keep doing what they studied, even if the medical system is doing things that don't go with their personal beliefs or medical ethics. You can't blame them, what else can they do? They have their hands tied and their mouths taped. This is definitely an unfortunate situation for the well meaning doctors and nurses.

The media and the government don't really want the public to know about all the corruption that takes place in big pharma and the CDC with all the negative vaccine side effects. A perfect example of this is the confession from CDC scientist, Dr William S Thompson, who was granted whistle blower status last February 2015 for putting out a statement to the government saying that he and his team omitted statistically significant information back in 2004 when the data was published in the journal of Pediatrics. The data that was omitted suggested that African American children younger than 36 months of age had a significantly higher risk of developing autism after receiving the MMR vaccine. This should be breaking news and the media should've spent hours talking and debating about this, but I bet you never heard about this. Do you know why? Because in my opinion, if the media brings this up as the biggest breaking news of the day or month, big pharma will stop their TV commercials on all the prescription medicine they advertise on TV every day, and that will hurt the profits of the networks. Don't forget that about 30% of the TV commercials are related to the latest pharmaceutical drugs. Think about it, why will you talk about negative issues from one of your main customers? If you do, your customers will leave. Conflict of interest? Yes, I think so.

Another example of big pharma corruption related to vaccines dates back to 2010 when two Merck virologists filed a federal lawsuit against Merck alleging that this drug company had lied about the effectiveness of the mumps vaccine. They claimed that Merck used improper testing methods, manipulated testing protocols, falsified test data, discarded undesirable test results and failed to report the actual low efficacy test results. Only recently, these virologists were given the green light to proceed with the lawsuit against Merck. It took the court system almost five years to agree and who knows how long it will take to actually go to trial and settle these claims. By the time they are allowed to go to court, the vaccine's patents will probably expire and Merck would've made billions of dollars in profit so paying 10-20 million dollars in settlement charges is a drop in a bucket for them.

Now let me tell you about corruption and lack of integrity at its best. Did you know that the most known pharmaceutical companies were managed by convicted Nazi operatives? Did you know that Hitler's government hired Bayer to make the poison gas that was used to kill Jews back in the 1940's?

As I mentioned earlier one of the best places to look for information about vaccines in general is the National Vaccine Information Center or NVIC, www.nvic.org. In this website you can find unbiased information regarding the latest news on any type of vaccines from the regular flu to the MMR recent exposures and failures. I follow this website because they are on top of the latest news and scientific studies. They are also a non-profit educational organization founded in 1982. They are 100% funded by donations. Their mission is to prevent vaccine injuries and deaths by educating the public to make informed decisions.

The current vaccination schedule calls for 49 doses of 14 vaccines by age 6. This is amazing because at this age, a child is in the early stages of development and their immune system gets shocked every time he/she gets injected with a vaccine. Vaccines are loaded with so many toxic ingredients that their small bodies react in many different ways. The medical system could at least spread the vaccine doses and start a little later than the current schedule. This has proven effective in countries that have made a change in some of the vaccines. For instance, Japan stopped using the MMR vaccine back in 1993 after 1.8 million children were given two types of MMR vaccines and a record number of children developed non-viral meningitis and many other adverse reactions. Today, Japan uses individual vaccines for measles, mumps and rubella.

Another example of vaccines in the United States and other countries is the relationship between infant mortality rate (IMR) and the number of vaccines before age 1. The US childhood immunization schedule calls for 26 doses for infants before they turn one year of age. This is the highest number of doses of any country in the world. The US also spends more money in health care cost than any country in the world; no one comes close – yet 33 other nations have lower IMR's than the US.

Statistical studies using regression analysis showed a high statistically significant correlation between the increased number of vaccine doses and an increase in infant mortality rates. Some countries have IMR's that are less than half the US rate. These countries are Japan, Sweden and Singapore. According to the CDC, the US IMR's appears to be worsening as the years pass. Premature deaths have increased in the United States by more than 20% between 1990 and 2006. How come no one talks about this? Why is it that the media only talks about a small outbreak in measles but no one talks about the infant mortality rates and other vaccine injuries? Well, we all know why based on what I explained earlier. As a point of reference, according to the CDC, as of April 3rd 2015, the total number of measles cases in the USA was only 159. Just to give you a broader perspective, this is equal to a super small percentage of 0.000049% in the US alone. Compare this small percentage with the number of deaths from FDA approved medicines which are more than 106 thousand people per year. By the way, so far in 2015 no one has died from measles and no one will probably die because the odds of this happening are very low.

An example of improper introduction of a vaccine is the Swine Flu vaccine during the big scare and big lie of a pandemic that never happened. For those of you who don't know, the swine flu vaccine was never properly approved. The FDA provided a waiver to allow big pharma to ship millions of this vaccine all over the United States and the world. To date the FDA has produced absolutely no scientific evidence documenting safety tests for the swine vaccine. There are no published studies, no records of any clinical trials, and no publicly-available paper trail demonstrating that any safety testing was done whatsoever. There is no researcher who has publicly put their name on the record declaring this vaccine to be safe, and no FDA official has ever stated that scientifically-valid safety testing has been conducted on this dangerous vaccine.

Most of the vaccines have not really been proven to be effective and their packaging inserts actually say this in clear English language; I'm not sure why the health officials purposely give a blind eye on this fact. An example of this fact is the Mumps outbreak of 2010 in New York and New Jersey. More than one thousand people got infected by this disease and according to the health authorities about 77% of those who caught mumps had already been vaccinated against this disease. I wonder if the person who admitted this to CNN is still employed; I seriously doubt it. Most of the people who had brought this up to the national media is somehow ridiculed or fired from their job for not properly filtering this type of information before it gets released to the national news networks.

Vaccines against infectious diseases don't really work. If they did, why do they still get sick when they get in contact with an infected person? If you are vaccinated, you should be 100% immunized right? Wrong. Even if you're given 3 or 4 booster shots, you're not even 90% safe from the disease. So, if this is the case, why get injected with a vaccine that has multiple side effects and the potential of killing you? Yes, killing you; if you don't believe me, read the paper they make you sign before they inject you with the vaccine. In fact, neither the CDC nor FDA can prove that the current vaccine schedule is safe. If vaccines are so safe, why do they make you sign a waiver? In fact, the next time you take your child to the doctor or hospital and they inform you that your child is due for another vaccine, ask the doctor or nurse to sign a document that says that they guarantee you 100% that the vaccine will not cause your child any harm what so ever and that they will be held responsible for any permanent injuries or death that the vaccine may cause. I'm sure you will be advised to search for another doctor because they will never sign it. But I don't blame the doctors or the thousands of clinics that administer vaccines for not signing such document because it is the pharmaceutical company that should be held responsible for any permanent damage or death. It is the vaccine maker that should be guaranteeing 100% the effectiveness of such vaccine. They should be signing such document, but unfortunately you will never get it signed and you will never be 100% safe with any of the vaccines that are currently forced to the public today.

Let's talk about the ingredients found in the most common vaccines. I cannot cover all the ingredients and their dangerous affects in this book because vaccines contain dozens of ingredients and it will take too long to cover all of them.

Vaccine ingredients can be divided into three main groups; Antigens, Adjuvants and Others including preservatives, precipitants and other chemicals.

Below are the most common ingredients found in vaccines.

Aluminum

This chemical has no benefit in the human body. It is categorized as a neurotoxin which means that it causes brain cell death. It is extremely toxic when mixed with mercury. This chemical has been shown to play a role in certain neurological diseases such as Alzheimer's, Autism, Parkinson's, seizures and even coma.

Antibiotics

These can affect the intestinal flora and can cause food allergies in some people. They deplete a very important antioxidant produced by the liver called Glutathione. They can cause hearing loss and allergic reactions ranging from mild to life threatening. They can also damage the kidneys.

Animal Cells

Yes, there are animal cells in vaccines. How would you like your child to get injected with animal cells? Not what you expected to hear, right? Some of the animal cells used in vaccines include calf fetus, chick embryo, chick kidney, cow heart, dog kidney, guinea pig embryo, horse blood, monkey brain cells, monkey kidney, chicken egg, duck egg, monkey lung, mouse blood, pig blood, rabbit brain and sheep blood among others. Some of these cells cause connective tissue disorders, chest pain, skin reactions, lupus and arthritis. Some of you may be thinking....ok, but we eat eggs and other animal products anyway, so what's the big deal? The difference is, when you eat these products your body digests, absorbs, filters and properly metabolizes those products while vaccines are injected directly into your blood stream and tissues with no chance of going through the same metabolic process. Besides, mouse blood, pig blood and monkey parts don't sound too appetizing to me and I'm sure you agree with me on this.

Human Aborted Fetal Tissue

If you believe in God and are Christian and you are against abortion, you should never allow your children to be injected with aborted fetal tissue. Most people don't know this but some vaccines are made with human aborted baby tissues. Such vaccines are Rubella in the MMR vaccine, Chicken Pox, Hepatitis-A, DTaP, Polio, Hib and Rabies. PER.C6 is a newer cell line developed by a company called Crucell and licensed by Merck. This patent says that the human embryonic retinoblast cells were isolated from the eyes of aborted fetuses of 18 to 21 weeks of age. Some people think this is okay but I don't. If you agree with me that vaccines should be made without the use of aborted tissues then ask questions and educate yourself about vaccines and their dangers. Don't turn a blind eye on such an important subject that may affect the life of your children. I don't ask you to believe me; I ask you to do your own research and make your own conclusions and decisions. The medical system doesn't own your children, so don't let them injure or cripple them for the rest of their lives. In my opinion, the new law in California signed by Governor Jerry Brown is unconstitutional because this law takes your religion freedom away from you as it mandates vaccines that promote abortion. The United States is mostly a Christian country but its people are misinformed about this and many other ingredients in food, medicines and personal products.

Detergents

These are cytotoxic and cause cells to leak or explode when they come in contact to the cell walls. This allows the vaccine ingredients to penetrate the cells more easily.

Formaldehyde

This is body embalming fluid used to preserve dead bodies. It is a colorless chemical also used in making building materials and household products. This is a well characterized poison. It is linked to leukemia, brain, colon and lymphatic cancer. It causes damage to the liver, nerve and reproductive system as well as the immune and respiratory system. It is ranked as one of the most hazardous chemicals to human health so why get injected with this poison?

Hydrocortisone

This is the synthetic form of cortisol which is the major stress hormone. This hormone can disrupt the development of infants and their endocrine function. It also affects the immune system, suppresses adrenal function and increases oxidative stress. Imagine shocking a human body with this ingredient at such an early age when the body is just developing. Common sense tells us this cannot be healthy to growing infants.

Sodium Borate

This chemical is also known as Borax and it is a neurotoxic not meant for internal use. Symptoms caused by this chemical include nausea, diarrhea, vomiting, respiratory and temperature changes, hyperactivity, mental confusion, shock, seizures, metabolic acidosis, vascular collapse and death. It may interfere with DNA and enzymes and it causes cell death.

Thimerasol

This is just another name for Mercury which is an extremely dangerous neurotoxin and carcinogen. This poison causes Autism in certain quantities. The problem is that it is very difficult to rid your body of mercury. It takes a special form of cleansing to remove it. There are about 25mcg of mercury in just one dose of the flu shot but the EPA (Environmental Protection Agency) claims that only 5mcg is safe. This means that children who receive multiple vaccines in one visit could be getting 10 times the EPA safety limit in just one day. Scary isn't it? if you have children, you should be scared and therefore you should educate yourself on this subject before they are harmed by medical system and be part of the VAERS statistics with minimum to no compensation. Read the form they make you sign and see all the side effects. As I said before, death is one of them. Why risk it?

These are just a few of the ingredients found in vaccines. Others include Antifungal, Benzethonium Chloride, Octoxynol 9, Sodium Deoxycholate, Sodium Taurodeoxycholate, Emulsifiers, Ethyl Green, Glutharaldehyde, Iron Ammonium Citrate, Phenoxyethanol, Phenol Red, Sorbitol, Sucrose, MSG and others.

Let's talk about the most common vaccines being administered today and pushed into the public, and their potential side effects. One of the biggest things people truly believe regarding vaccines is that they are scientifically tested by the FDA and hence fully approved by FDA scientists. Nothing can be further from the truth. One of the first questions you should be asking is, what kind of studies have been conducted to make sure vaccines are safe? Also, what are the scientific proof and evidence that vaccines are completely safe for infants, pregnant women, small children and the elderly who are the most vulnerable? How about the safety of those with asthma or patients with compromised immune systems? All this has to be taken in consideration and properly studied before getting injected with a potentially hazardous vaccine. Wouldn't you like to make sure your children are ready for the vaccine? Wouldn't you do anything to make sure your children are safe? Of course you would and that's why you should spend some time educating yourself so you can ask the doctor or nurse the right questions before accepting the vaccine. Don't rely on the nurse telling you not to worry about the side effects or the minor fever your child may develop. Remember, they are human beings and they also make mistakes. They also don't have the time to keep current on all the independent studies that suggest that vaccines are extremely dangerous. They also don't know about all the medical doctors who used to believe in vaccines and now are totally against them. Please don't gamble with your life and read more about this subject. It is a very important step to keep yourself and your children safe from the dangers of vaccines. If you decide to continue allowing the medical system experiment with your body and that of your children even after doing your homework, that's fine because it is your own decision based on your own research. Don't do it only because that's the way it has been since the early 1950's; do it because you believe it is best for your children. The key here is education. Please read the book "A shot in the Dark" by Doctor Harris L Coulter and Barbara Loe Fisher. Or "Saying No to Vaccines" by Dr Sherri Tenpenny. Or "Vaccines, Autism and Childhood Disorders" by Neil Z Miller. There are many books on this subject written by medical doctors who used to think vaccines were the way to go and now are speaking about the risks and potential permanent damage of vaccines.

Please don't be alarmed by this chapter because as I said before, every human body is different and all of us react differently to medicines and vaccines. Not every child will be affected the same way so if you choose to vaccinate your children please talk to their pediatrician and ask him/her if it's possible to delay a vaccine or at least spread them in different months or years so the risk is minimized. They should be totally okay with this suggestion. Also, please make sure their immune system is strong by feeding them healthy foods that nourish their bodies. A strong immune system is their best defense so as a parent you should be doing everything possible to feed them the right foods.

I hope this short chapter of the book has given you some food for thought on this subject and provided you with the tools needed to discuss it with your doctor and continue your research on this very important life changing subject.

Vaccines summary

- Vaccines are highly dangerous

- They have never been proven effective. You are the guinea pig

- Hygiene, drinking water and good nutrition are 700% more effective than vaccines

- Most vaccines have mercury (Thimerosal), aluminum, formaldehyde, antibiotics, MSG and animal cells

- The documentation that comes with vaccines says there is no clear correlation between the presence of an antibody and protection against a disease. In short, they don't really work

- About 11,300 newborns die within 24 hours of their birth in the United States each year. That's 50% more first day deaths than all other industrialized countries combined. In the US Hepatitis B vaccine is given to newborns within hours of being born. Why can't they wait until the baby is at least 1 year old? Some countries do.

- Infant mortality is higher in the US than in 35 other industrialized countries. US had one of the best rates before vaccines were mandatory.

- In 1985 only 33 vaccines were recommended before entering kindergarten. In 2008, this figure rose to 113 before kindergarten and 150 by 11th grade. Autism rates have also risen, is there a link? maybe

- Less than 15% of the world population got the smallpox vaccine. The disease disappeared thanks to drinking water, hygiene and sanitation. US reported no cases of Smallpox since 1950. Vaccinations were stopped in 1971.

- The Polio disease was almost eradicated when the Polio vaccine was implemented in 1954. Again, I believe hygiene, sanitation and better drinking water did most of the job

- There are still 10 to 11 countries that have problems with Polio today. Parts of these countries have no drinking water, no sewers and no toilets. Hygiene conditions are terrible. Could that be the reason? I think so

- Those who receive the recommended 6 doses of the Measles vaccines (MMR) may be 3 times more likely to acquire Crohn's disease (inflammation of the digestive tract)

- Studies in England suggest that the MMR vaccine (Measles, Mumps and Rubella) is associated with a high number of Arthritis

- Pharmaceutical companies have been using tissues from aborted babies since 1960 to develop some vaccines

- Vaccines made with tissues from aborted babies are: Rubella in the MMR vaccine, Chicken Pox, Hepatitis-A, DTaP, Polio, Hib and Rabies

- A study of the Clinic for Infectious Diseases concluded that all cases of polio in the US since 1980 were caused by the Polio vaccine. If you are not outraged by now, I don't know what will

- A study of the Clinic for Infectious Disease confirms that the DPT (Diphtheria, Pertussis and Tetanus) vaccine induces or causes polio. Unbelievable, don't you think?

- In the 1950's and 1960's, millions of people were injected with polio vaccines that were contaminated with the SV-40 virus (African green monkeys infected with AIDS). So AIDS may have been caused by an error from the health authorities. Do you still trust them?

- In 1979 Japan ordered to postpone the Pertussis vaccine from 2 months to 2 years of age. The result was the complete elimination of Sudden Infant Death Syndrome SIDS. Why doesn't the US follow suit?

- An epidemic of whooping cough in Cincinnati, affected hundreds of children, 75% of whom already had several Pertussis vaccines. I bet you only heard 5 seconds of this on the news. But the CDC still pushes for this vaccine even though it may not protect your child from the disease.

- Dr. Roy Anderson of the University of Oxford, says that vaccines are the most dangerous weapons of medicine and they may cause an inevitable human mutation

- In 1986 the "National Childhood Vaccine Injury Act" was signed into law. This law says that no one can sue a doctor, clinic or pharmaceutical company for any damages caused by any vaccine. So, if your child dies because of the vaccine, no one goes to jail. Sorry.

- Over $1.4 Billion dollars have been paid to families who now have children with permanent damage or have died from vaccines

- There are more than 5,000 outstanding cases of autistic children today, possibly caused by the vaccines

- VAERS is a government database that holds all the adverse events caused by vaccines. Unfortunately, according to the FDA and the CDC, only 10% of these adverse cases are reported by doctors. It is believed that less than 25% of people are compensated because it is very difficult to verify that the vaccine actually cause the adverse reaction or death

- Records from US Congress (2000-2003) indicate that pharmaceutical companies care more about the profits than people's safety. This is no surprise since they were given criminal immunity by the government back in 1986 as I explained earlier.

- Measles declined 95% in the US between 1915 and 1958. The vaccine was introduced in 1963. The medical establishment claims the vaccine eradicated the disease when in fact it was already 95% eradicated. In fact, post-vaccination death rates for measles in the mid 1970's are similar to those of the pre-vaccination years in the early 1960's when the vaccine was instituted.

- Chickenpox is not a life threatening illness and has no serious complications. Vaccination is considered unnecessary by many authorities. The American Academy of Pediatrics (AAP) as late as 1996 indicated in its immunization brochure that "Most children who are otherwise healthy and get chickenpox won't have any complications from the disease". This vaccine was added to the schedule in 1995.

- Hepatitis B: The risk of infants contracting this disease is close to non-existent. This vaccine may be appropriate for people of high risk such as prostitutes and IV drug addicts such as heroin users and others. This vaccine is injected to newborns shortly after birth, many times without parent's consent. This is a calamity in my opinion.

- HPV vaccine: There are over 100 HPV strains and about 30 of them are transmitted sexually. In rare occasions 10 of these viruses may cause cancer. The drug Gardasil only targets 4 of these. The problem is that this drug hasn't been proven to actually prevent cancer. Most women who get HPV clears it from the system naturally as long as their immune system is not compromised. Gardasil increases the incident of fever by 1,400% and vomiting by 1,500%.

Documented side effects in medical literature and vaccine pamphlets

- Arthritis

- Allergies

- Blood clots

- Septicemia

- Heart attacks

- Ear infections

- Sudden Infant Death Syndrome (SIDS)

- Epilepsy, autism

- Fainting

- Kidney disease

- Liver Diseases

- Severe allergic reactions

- Neurological problems

- Immunological diseases

- Fever, headache and muscle ache

- Serious reactions including death

How to Identify a Vaccine Reaction

- High fever (over 103F)

- High pitched screaming

- Joint pain

- Skin (hives, rashes, swelling)

- Collapse or shock, been unresponsive

- Excessive sleeping

- Convulsions

- Loss of muscle control

- Paralysis

- Brain inflammation

- Encephalopathy or brain damage

- Sudden death

THE MIRACLES OF HERBS

Natural herbs and some vegetables are perhaps the first natural "medicines" that we should use for a mild illness such as headache, fever or even stress. Unfortunately the first thing that most people do is reach for the medicine cabinet and take either prescription drugs or over the counter medicines. This has been classified as an epidemic in the US not only because television advertisements are flooded with commercials about medicines but also because it seems that there is a pharmacy on every corner. On top of this, almost every supermarket in the US has its own pharmacy. This creates an easy pathway for people to self prescribe medicines that sometimes cause death. Remember that more than one hundred thousand people die each year in the US by taking fully approved FDA drugs.

Natural herbs may be the answer to many illnesses. In fact they are so effective that pharmaceutical companies have produced countless medicines based on certain herbs or spices. The problem is, these companies cannot patent an herb so they make a synthetic form of the herb and add a bunch of ingredients and chemicals to mass produce it and patent it so they can make billions of dollars. In this part of the book I'll explain which herbs are the most effective for different diseases and pain. In Latin America, the indigenous have used herbs for many years with amazing results. The sad thing is that the medical system in most developed countries do not accept any claims or healing powers of natural herbs because they are not part of a controlled scientific study. I understand that curative claims must be made in a controlled manner to ensure its effectiveness and validity. There is nothing wrong with regulating that aspect. However, I can assure you that no pharmaceutical company would accept the challenge to compare one of their drugs face to face with an herb that has certain healing powers of a given disease. I dare to say that it is very likely that in the long term the herb would be more effective than the drug being compared and with no negative side effects. The marketing of FDA approved drugs is huge in the US and that is probably the main reason most people are used to taking them. In the US is very common to see drug commercials in almost all television channels. These commercials begin with a dramatization of the pain and suffering caused by a certain illness and then it explains the supposed benefit of such medicine. At the end, they explain the side effects of these medicines. My family and I laugh at the negative side effects each time they show those commercials. The side effects are so dangerous and horrendous that we often question…..Who in their right mind is going to buy a medicine that causes cancer or death? Unfortunately many people watch those commercials and never pay attention to the side effects and when they go to the doctor they demand a prescription for one of those drugs from a TV commercial.

In earlier civilizations, medicine and food were intimately connected. Many of the plants were eaten for their healing powers. The Egyptians, for example, used garlic to ward off epidemics that existed at the time of the pyramids. The two current civilizations that still employ the use of herbology are India and China. Medicinal plants are used as part of a therapeutic system in India. This therapy is known worldwide as Ayurvedic medicine. In most of the Chinese hospitals, they use the traditional modern medicine along with Chinese Medicine with great success. Chinese medicine is known worldwide for being a natural therapy with great benefits. In many countries it is very common to find doctors of Chinese medicine (including the US) since it is recognized and named as an ancient medicine with positive results.

Chinese medicine is an ancient system of healing. This was born over 2,000 years ago and is based on the philosophy that people perceive balances and imbalances within themselves and their surroundings. This medicine views disease in terms of patterns of disharmony and seeks to establish a balance in the sick person. It is believed that the energy flows through channels called meridians.

There are many books related to this alternative medicine with details on each of their natural herbs. If you are interested in this alternative medicine I advise you to do more research on this topic. In this book I only explain a small part of its importance.

Herbs and vegetables in Central and South America

This continent is full of plants and flowers with amazing magical healing powers. The use of medicinal spiritual plants by ancient civilizations is legendary and recognized worldwide. The Aztecs who dominated Central America in the past, had a wide knowledge of the healing powers of plants. When the Spaniards conquered Mexico in the sixteenth century they discovered more than 1,200 medicinal plants.

The doctors of the Maya medicine are still masters of spiritual medicine plants and used plants to connect with the spirits of nature which provides them with the vision of other medicinal plants.

In Machu Picchu, Peru, the Incas used to gather in ceremonies and rituals with coca leaves. These rituals are extremely important in the Inca civilization and the Q'ueros who still live in the mountains around the city of Cuzco. They believe in the balance and energy created by Mother Nature and their spiritual and healing powers which this provides.

Let's talk about each of the most important herbs and vegetables according to the leading experts in the field. As I said before, I cannot provide you with all the herbs and their healing powers in this book because it will require more than 500 pages to list them all. The intention of this part of the book is to give you short but vital information to educate you about the healing powers of these herbs.

Garlic (Latin - Allium sativum)

It is believed that garlic comes from central Asia. Garlic is known worldwide and for centuries for its healing powers. It is one of the oldest medicinal plants of our planet. As I explained before the Egyptians used garlic to stay away from epidemics and gave it to the slaves in the days of the pyramids. Garlic has antibiotic and antiseptic powers. It has expectorant properties, it is a fungicide and an anti-histamine. If consumed regularly it can prevent influenza, flu and ear infections. It can also help with mucus and coughing as well as intestinal worms and fungal infections. It is a very powerful lung cleanser that helps relieve asthma attacks. If eaten with foods or as a natural oil, garlic can help with circulation, reduces blood clots, blood pressure and lowers cholesterol. It is also very beneficial for thrombosis patients. But perhaps the most important and beneficial power of garlic is its ability to cure and prevent cancer. This was recognized by Hippocrates in the fourth century BC.

Aloe (Latin – Aloe communis)

This section is dedicated to Dilia Florez Rojas as she was the first person who bought and read the Spanish version of this book in its entirety and her only comment she had for me was the fact that I didn't have a section about Aloe and its amazing powers. I agree with her and hence I am including this section in her honor. She is now in heaven looking after all of us. Rest in peace. We love you Dilia and thank you for your feedback.

Aloe is native to the South and East Africa. Native Indians call aloe leaves "Magic wands from heaven" for its healing powers. The healing powers of aloe have been written and recognized for centuries and has been used by many civilizations. The positive effects of this plant are countless and priceless. Aloe is rich in many vitamins such as vitamin C, B1, B2 and B6. It is also rich in calcium, potassium, enzymes, natural sugars and contains more than 16 amino acids. When this is applied to the skin, it helps to regenerate healthy cells. Another important use of this plant for the skin is for relieving sunburn, acne and eczema. Aloe vera can be taken with fruit juices, smoothies or by itself. When ingested, aloe vera juice helps with digestive and gastro-intestinal problems. Aloe vera is a plant with anti fungal, anti-inflammatory and antiseptic powers. Most people believe that aloe can only be used in a topical form for burns. The truth is that aloe has a lot of internal uses of great importance for overall human health.

According to Mike Adams, editor and founder of naturalnews.com, aloe is the most impressive medicinal herb that Mother Nature has created. He says garlic is the second best. This plant has been studied over the years and is known as a plant that can stop the growth of cancerous tumors since it helps raise the immune system. It also helps lower cholesterol and triglycerides, repairs and reverses sticky blood from the arteries due to glucose, increases blood oxygenation, reduces inflammation and relieves arthritis pain, prevents kidney stones, alkalizes the blood, heals ulcers, Crohn's disease and other digestive disorders. Lowers blood pressure, helps stop colon cancer, lubricates the digestive tract and the intestines, eliminates constipation, prevents and relieves Candida infections. It can be used as a sports drink because it contains a good balance of electrolytes. Increases cardiovascular performance and endurance. Hydrates the skin and accelerates skin repair.

Aloe has a phyto-nutrient called Acemannan, which has anti-cancer powers and raises the immune system. In a study with dogs and cats that were being exposed to radiation, the group of animals that were given acemannan during and after radiation had a significantly higher tumor reduction than the group that was not given acemannan.

What does it contain?

Water, 20 Minerals, 12 Vitamins, 18 Amino-acids, Fito-nutrients, Enzymes, Triterpens (lowers glucose leves), Glico-nutrients and Glico-proteins, Polisacarides (Acemannan, Mannose-6-Phosphate).

How to Prepare it

Remove the skin and fillet the inner gelatinous portion. Use this material to make juices and smoothies. If this is the first time you take aloe I suggest you start with a small amount as this can have a laxative effect at first. Enjoy this miraculous plant and tell your friends and family to enjoy their curative and digestive powers. If it helps you, say a prayer for Dilia please.

Cayenne Pepper (Latin – Capsicum Minimum)

Cayenne pepper has been used for many years for therapeutic purposes. This spice has powerful anti-inflammatory effects, stimulates circulation and neutralizes acidity in the body. It has the ability to relieve ulcers, stomach pain, sore throat, spasmodic cough and helps relieve diarrhea. This spice has been used for different kinds of diseases such as Gout, Acid reflux, Delirium, Paralysis, Fever, Atonic dyspepsia, Hemorrhoids, Nausea, Tonsillitis and Diphtheria. During a cold or flu, cayenne pepper helps move the congested mucus. There have been several studies on this spice and they indicate that the cayenne pepper is very effective in preventing the formation of fungal pathogens. Remember that cancer is a fungus and therefore pepper can be very effective for reducing cancer tumors. In one study, scientists demonstrated an 80% reduction of prostate cancer in rats. The capsaicin in cayenne pepper helps destroy cancer cells by themselves. Pepper contains many beneficial phytochemicals as well as vitamin C, E and minerals including magnesium which is extremely vital for heart health. It cleanses the blood helping hormonal signals flow easily through the blood stream to enhance the immune system.

Onion (Allium cepa)

Comes from Asia but for thousands of years it is grown in subtropical regions in several parts of the world. Onions contain volatile essences and possess a unique spicy flavor. In kitchens it is popular for its characteristic to make you cry. This is because the volatile essences enter the nose causing the well known tearing. Another well known but undesirable characteristic of the onion is that is causes bad breath for several hours after ingestion, especially when eaten raw. Onion is one of the healthiest and most impressive healing plants. It has a high content of vitamin A, B, C and E and for its generous content of vitamin C, onion raises the immune system and therefore increases the body's defenses.

These are some of the nutritional properties that are found in a single 100 gram onion. Water - 86g, carbohydrates - 10g, fat - 0.2g, potassium - 180 mg, Sulphur - 70mg, Phosphorus - 44mg, Calcium - 32mg, Vitamin C - 28mg, Magnesium - 16mg, Sodium - 7 mg, Iron - 0.5mg, Manganese - 0.25mg, Zinc - 0.08mg and others of less value.

Benefits of onion

Onions are rich in minerals and its high content of vitamins A and C makes it an essential plant for the possible treatment and cure of respiratory diseases. It also helps protect the body from parasites and infections. Its properties of iron, phosphorus and other minerals are important for the treatment of anemia.
Onions are also used to treat diseases such as rheumatism, diabetes, obesity, asthma, nervousness, tuberculosis, diarrhea, bronchial and bladder diseases, arthritis, the flu, cough, insomnia, bleeding, sore throat, prostate issues, minor skin infections, headache and earache, rhinitis and chronic colds.

As you can see onions are of paramount importance and can be consumed daily, either raw or cooked in low heat. The greatest nutritional value is in its raw form because heat reduces some of the nutritional powers.

Ginkgo (Ginkgo Biloba)

This is known as the most ancient medicinal plant as the Ginkgo tree comes from the age of the dinosaurs. A Ginkgo tree can live to be a thousand years and it is well known all over the world for its powers to enhance and extend life. It is an elixir of youth and science has shown that the leaves are super rich in quercetin and catechin tannis which are substances that increase blood supply and oxygenation of the tissues. Studies have shown that Ginkgo can be used as an herbal medicine to reduce age related memory loss. It may also help with atherosclerosis, vertigo and impotence. The Ginkgo tree can grow to amazing heights reaching about 180 feet and the leaves are fan shaped. It is considered the oldest tree on earth and it is considered sacred by many Far East cultures.

Cinnamon (Cinnamomum Verum)

Cinnamon is considered a treasured spice and it is one of the most popular remedies in China to treat winter cold, sore throat and coughs. If you have bad breath, you can chew a stick of cinnamon; it can also aid in the digestion after meals. In the ancient Egyptian times, cinnamon was used to ward off infections and for embalming. If you have type 2 diabetes, eating only half a teaspoon daily can help you reduce blood glucose levels dramatically. That's not all, cinnamon has also been proven to reduce total cholesterol, triglycerides and LDL or bad cholesterol. This incredible spice also helps ward off urinary tract infections. When you buy cinnamon, make sure you get the sticks that have layers on them because the ones that are a solid stick are not real cinnamon. Those are called "Cassia". The real kind is called "Ceylon". They don't come from the same plant but they both offer an anticoagulant property. Most of the ground cinnamon sold in stores come from cassia.

Cardamon (Elattaria Cardamomum)

This plant grows wild in the monsoon forest of southern India and Sri Lanka. This is one of the most ancient culinary spices in the world. This spice is known in India as grains of paradise and the seeds are valued for their medicinal properties. It is used by the Hindu system of Ayurvedic medicine. The Egyptians also added cardamom to their religious ceremonies and even Hippocrates in Greece, embraced it due to its exquisite aroma and therapeutic powers.

Fig (Ficus Carica)

The fig is the first fruit mentioned in the bible and it is believed to be one of the healthiest fruit. Figs are thought to have been first cultivated in Egypt. In ancient Greece they became a staple foodstuff in the traditional diet. In ancient Rome they were thought of as a sacred fruit. It is a good source of potassium which helps control blood pressure. It is also a good source of fiber, vitamin B6, copper, manganese and pantothenic acid. In some cultures, fig leaves are part of the menu. The leaves have been shown to have anti-diabetic properties and can reduce the amount of insulin needed by diabetics. In one study, a liquid extract made from fig leaves was added to the breakfast of insulin dependent diabetics to produce an insulin lowering effect. In animal studies, fig leaves have been shown to reduce levels of triglycerides and in in-vitro studies its leaves inhibited the growth of certain types of cancer cells. People with existing and untreated kidney and gallbladder problems should avoid eating figs because they contain oxalates which can crystallize and cause health issues when they become too concentrated in body fluids.

St. John's Wort (Hypericum Perforatum)

This herb is very popular and can be acquired in many different forms over the counter. It is used to treat mild depression and there is some scientific evidence that suggests it might be effective for treating anxiety and menopausal symptoms. There are however a few precautions for this herb. One of the active ingredients is a compound known as photoactive hypericins which produce substances that can damage cells when the skin is exposed to sunlight. There is a fatty insulation that wraps around nerves called myelin; this insulation is particularly vulnerable to the damage caused by sunlight. For this reason, food based supplements like Triptophan is a preferred substitute for mild depression and anxiety. Mayo Clinic has additional safety information for people with known allergy or sensitivity to this herb and its parts; some of them include infrequent allergic skin reactions, including rash and itching. This herb may also increase the risk of serotonin syndrome, may change how sugar is processed in the body so use with caution if you are diabetic. It may cause high levels of thyroid stimulating hormone (TSH). Use with caution if you have cataracts and are prone to swelling. It may damage the liver, alter blood pressure and increase heart rate. There are many more potential risks associated with this herb. For a complete list of side effects of this herb please go to www.mayoclinic.org. As I said before, every person is different and this herb may not affect everyone the same way. In fact, this herb may be very beneficial to some people so please do your research on this herb and listen to your body each time you take it to know if it helps you or not. Education is the key to everything and this is no exception.

Tee Tree (Malaleuca Alternifolia)

This powerful plant is found in Australia and it has been used by native aborigines for centuries. Tee Tree is a cousin to eucalyptus and belongs to the family of paperbark trees that have a strong medicinal scent. The aborigines used it to make small canoes, knife sheaths and thatches for shelters. They used the leaves to make medicine to treat colds, coughs and headaches. Tea tree is well known for its antiseptic properties and can be used as an antibiotic for small external infections including minor ear infections. You can also make an infusion of its leaves and use it as a mouthwash, to apply on the skin to treat acne and spray it on children's head for keeping head lice at bay. Adding 8-10 drops of tea tree essential oil to the bath twice a week can boost resistance to many types of infections.

Tea tree has been documented in many medical and scientific studies because it has been proven to kill bacteria, fungi and viruses. Back in the 1940's tea tree was known as the antiseptic medicine to have at all times. Australian WWII soldiers were given tea tree in their first aid kits. There are more than 300 scientific studies that talk about the antimicrobial powers of teat tree. Here is a list of illnesses and infections that tea tree is effective for treatment: Acne, cold sores, earaches, head lice, bacterial infections, respiratory tract infections, chickenpox, halitosis (bad breath), psoriasis, MRSA and itchy insect bites among others. At home, it can also serve as an acne face wash, insect repellant, deodorant, to removes, to remove foot odor, as a laundry freshener and as a household cleaner. Many doctors of functional medicine prescribe essential oils like teat tree oil and coconut oil as replacement for conventional medicines because these don't have any adverse side effects and are just as effective.

Olive (Olea europaea)

Olive has been regarded as sacred for centuries in southern Europe. In ancient Greece it was worshiped as Athena, the goddess of wisdom and learning. In Judaism, olive oil is considered holy and it is used as fuel for the Sabbath lamp and for the menorah in the festival of Hanukkah. Olives are considered one of the richest sources of vitamin E. There are many types of olive oils to choose from in the market place; cold-pressed olives are the best to produce good quality virgin oil. It is rich in monounsaturated fatty acids and it plays an important role in protecting the heart and circulatory system. Olive oil and macadamia oil are Omega 9 fatty acids in the form of oleic acid. These are considered non essential oils because the body can create them from unsaturated fats. However, the standard American diet contains saturated fats, processed foods and GMO foods which inhibit the body from producing these Omega 9 fatty acids. Adding olive oil to your diet is therefore very important in my opinion and that of many experts. In different parts of Europe doctors recommend olives to diabetics and people with liver problems. It is also used in Chinese medicine to relieve sore throats. Olive oil softens the skin and helps restore luster to dull hair. There are three well known Omega fatty acids, Omega 3, 6 and 9. There should be a balance of all three and especially Omega 3 and 6. According to the experts, the ideal ratio of Omega 3 to Omega 6 fats should be 1:1. However, the typical American diet has a ratio between 1:20 and 1:40 in some cases. This means that the average American is consuming far too many polyunsaturated fats and way too little Omega 3 fats. This is a very dangerous ratio and the balance should be tipped over to the proper ratio before it's too late. No wonder why heart disease is the number one cause of death in the United States and most Western societies. The body needs the right ratio of these essential fatty acids to be at its optimum state. Omega 6 fats stimulate inflammation processes instead of inhibiting them. The body needs some inflammation to protect itself from infections and trauma and a certain amount of polyunsaturated fats help protect the body. However, consuming too much of these fats increases chronic inflammation which causes many health problems over the long term. There is a great article in doctor Mercola's website www.mercola.com which talks about all these fats. He explains in plain English the differences between saturated, unsaturated, monounsaturated and polyunsaturated fats. Visit this website for a thorough understanding of these fats. I will give you a quick summary here. **Saturated fats** – These are fully loaded with hydrogen atoms and are typically solid at room temperature. **Unsaturated fats-** These are fats that have lost at least one of their pairs of hydrogen atoms which result in molecules that bend at each double bond. These fats come in two varieties - **Monounsaturated** which are missing one pair of hydrogen atoms and **Polyunsaturated** which are missing more than one pair of hydrogen atoms.

Ginseng (Panax Quinquefolius and P Ginseng)

There are two types of ginseng, Asian and American ginseng. They have different benefits and Chinese medicine considers American ginseng less stimulating than the Asian variety. Ginseng is mostly known in Asia as an elixir of life. It represents strength, vigor and virility. This plant and herb is used to boost mood, improve memory and attention, lengthen physical and mental endurance and ease anxiety. It also boosts concentration and focus when combined with Ginkgo. Some studies have found that ginseng may boost the immune system. Several studies also suggest that ginseng may lower blood sugar levels. Ginseng has also been studied to treat cancer, high blood pressure, hepatitis C, fatigue, heart disease and erectile dysfunction. There are no natural foods that contain ginseng and hence it is very important that you buy this herb from reputable companies or health food stores. This is an expensive root so if you see low prices been advertised, be very cautious because the ingredients, quality and potency may not be the most optimal or may be adulterated ginseng.

In the Far East ginseng has always been the ultimate cure-all herb that prolongs life and enhances physical stamina. Chinese and Vietnamese troops are said to carry a root so that they are alert to danger and increase their physical activity. In Chinese medicine it is seen as a medicine that restores balance in a stressed and strained body. The Asiatic ginseng is good for body building and endurance sports, while the American variety targets the nervous system, improves memory and learning. It also prevents circulatory problems and blood clotting which in turn reduces the risk of stroke.

There you have it. There are many more herbs and plants but I can't cover all of them in this book. I hope you can reap from the benefits of these herbs and plants and implement some of them in your daily diet. If you are interested about this subject and would like more information, you can visit doctor Mercola's website.

SUMMARY

Dear reader, I hope this book gives you the tools needed to live a long healthy life without having to worry about viruses floating around or your co-worker infecting you during the flu season.

It is my hope that this book has helped you to consider adding exercise and healthy eating habits to your daily routine to nourish your temple, your body. Understanding healthy eating, nutrition and exercise are the basis for disease prevention.

In my opinion, if you follow at least 85% of the recommendations in this book, it is very likely that your immune system will get stronger and your nutrition level will increase tenfold. Remember that the father of western medicine, Hippocrates, said that food should be your medicine. There is no medicine in the world that can cure a disease 100%; No doctor can deny this or claim otherwise. Medicine only treat the symptom instead of mitigating the root cause and curing the disease. Only your own body has the ability to heal itself, but the body needs your help by providing it with healthy and nutritious food and avoiding junk food, processed food and any other food made in a lab. Conventional medicine is not the solution to most diseases or pain. Health care in the US (or sick care as I call it) is based on the promise that you can be healed and treated temporarily instead of actually curing the disease. The problem is that most FDA approved drugs have dozens of side effects that have much higher risks than the benefits they claim and promise. These side effects become a vicious cycle of other drugs that cause other diseases. In many cases the side effects are so severe that they cause permanent damage to the liver and other vital organs. Most of the time the patient is unaware that the new disease was caused by the medicine that he or she was taking for a different disease. In this book I provided you with several suggestions to help you make a change in your diet and life style. Many of these suggestions may help you prevent and possibly cure most chronic diseases. As I mentioned, these diseases generate billions of dollars to a hand full of multi-national corporations. With these recommendations you now have the opportunity to make your own decision to change your life and that of others in your friends and family circle to live a healthier life. Do not ignore the reality of the current health statistics and please do not wait for a miracle to happen when you are in your 70's because it may be too late to reverse any disease you may have at that point.

Before you make any changes to your diet, it is recommended by many experts to do a liver and colon cleanse to detoxify these very important organs to help you achieve a faster healthier you. As I explained in the juicing chapter, the best way to do a detox is by engaging in a liquid/juicing diet for at least 5-7 days. This is the safest and most effective way of ridding your body of toxins according to the experts on this subject like Dr Joe Mercola, Dr Brian Clement of the Hippocrates Health Institute, Dr Max Gurson and others. You can also use some supplements to do a cleanse but please be careful with supplements because they may cause some other issues. If you choose that route, look for food based supplements from well known health food stores instead of large retail stores. Juicing is my favorite and I recommend it because your body will feel the change on the fourth day with side effects like weight loss, healthy glowing skin, more energy and elimination of craving for the wrong foods.

It is your choice to be or not to be part of the horrible US health care statistics, or should I say "sick care statistics". I know it's not easy to stop the bad habits of unhealthy foods, smoking and others due to the convenience and very inexpensive food choices at the fast food restaurants. Perhaps you can start with small changes in your diet and gradually incorporate healthier choices until your body switches the cravings from the wrong foods to healthier ones. I guarantee you that once you start to notice positive results, you will want to make changes faster so you can enjoy life without pain or disease. But the best feeling of all is to know that you can stop thinking that you may be a victim of the death statistics that are currently robbing people from being able to live 15, 20 and even 30 years longer. No one likes to hear the bad news that you have diabetes or cancer so why not do something to prevent these diseases. Why not invest in your health early on so you can enjoy the benefits later in life when your body starts to age?

Think about this and do it for your children or grandchildren or simply to feel good and live life like it's meant to be lived. Believe me, you will have more energy, vitality and an elevated mood that you probably haven't had for many years. You will notice changes in the skin because the skin is an outward expression of your interior. I hope you join me in my mission to advocate health and prevention to all your friends and family so together we can save a person's life or at least help that person understand the dangers of pharmaceutical drugs and their side effects.

Remember that before making changes in your diet or start an exercise routine you should consult your general practitioner. Even though most of them don't really know much about nutrition and prevention through healthy eating, I need to say this for legal purposes.

I leave for now but I want you to know that I will continue to educate myself and will continue to be a health advocate to educate others on the importance of prevention through healthy eating. I will also persist with this message through other books in the near future. Remember what the father of modern medicine, Hippocrates, said "Let food be thy medicine". So eat well and let your body heal itself with good nutrition.

Thanks for taking the time to read this information and for allowing me to communicate all the research that I've compiled in this book. May God be always on your side protecting your health and that of your family.

APPENDIX

Mercury Levels in Fish
(Average in parts per million or PPM)

Species	Average	Species	Average
Tilefish	1.45	Carp	0.11
Shark	0.99	Whitefish	0.09
Sword fish	0.97	Squid	0.07
King Mackerel	0.73	Crab	0.06
Marlin	0.49	Pollock	0.06
Tuna	0.38	Catfish	0.05
Tuna (Albacore)	0.35	Red Mullet	0.05
Snook	0.35	Scallops	0.05
Blue fish	0.31	Herring	0.04
Lobster	0.31	Haddock	0.03
Bass	0.27	Trout	0.03
Halibut	0.26	River crab	0.03
Sea Trout	0.25	Crawfish	0.03
Turbot	0.24	Anchovies	0.02
Red Snapper	0.19	Sardines	0.02
Monkfish	0.18	Salmon	0.01
Sea Snook	0.15	Tilapia	0.01
Perch	0.14	Oysters	0.01
Tuna (Light)	0.12	Clam	0.01
Cod	0.11	Shrimp	0.01

Adapted from EPA/FDA data. FDA testing is very limited and may not reflect actual contamination levels

Acidic Foods

Acidic Foods
- White flour (bleached white flour)
- White rice, salt, white sugar
- Cereals with artificial sugars and flavors
- White refined pasta
- Prescription and over the counter medications
- Beer (pH 2.5) - Hard liquor - Wine - Cigarettes
- Meats (beef, pork, chicken)
- Bacon - Lamb - Rabbit - Turkey - Veal - Venison
- Lobster - Clams - Haddok - Mussels - Oyster - Shrimp
- Salmon - Sardines - Sausage -Scallops - Tuna - Cod
- Processed meats - Eggs - Cows milk cheese
- Microwavable foods - Vinegar - Yeast
- Pasteurazied and homogenized milk
- Coffee (pH 4.0) - Cafeinated drinks - Sodas (pH 2.0)
- Peanuts - Pecans - Walnuts - Tahini
- Milk chocolate
- Mermelade - Jelly - Honey
- Mustard - Ketchup - Mayonaise - Butter
- Green plaintains
- Blueberries - Rasberries - Cranberries
- Currants - Canned or glazed fruits
- Corn - Soda crackers - Cornstarch - Macaroni
- Wheat germ - Rye - Rice cakes - Quinoa - Kamut

Alkaline Foods

Alkalizing Foods
- Alfalfa - Barley grass - Beet greens - Beets - Carrots - Celery
- Broccoli - Cauliflower - Cabage - Chard greens - Cucumber
- Chlorella - Dandelions - Eggplant - Garlic - Green beens - Kale
- Green peas - Lettuce - Mushrooms - Mustard greens - Onions
- Parsnips - Peas - Peppers - Pumpkin - Radishes - Sea veggies
- Spinach - Green spirulina - Sprouts - Tomatoes - Watercress
- Sweet potatoes - Wheat grass - Wild greens - Kombu - Nori
- Daikon - Maitake - Wakame - Reishi - Shitake - Umeboshi
- Kelp - Mango - Cayene - Papaya - Parsley - Seaweeds - Kiwi
- Asparagus - Passionfruit - Avocado - Bell peppers
- Apple - Apricot - Avocado - Banana (high glycemic)
- Blackberries - Cantaloupe - Cherries - Coconut - Dates - Figs
- Grapes - Grapefruit - Honeydew melon - Lemon - Lime - Pear
- Nectarine - Orange - Peach - Pineapple - Raisins - Raspberries
- Strawberries - Tangerine - Watermelon - Tropical fruits
- Almonds - Chestnuts - Millet - Tempeh - Tofu (fermented)
- Stevia - Chili pepper - Cinnamon - Curry - Ginger - Miso - Herbs
- Sea salt - Tamari - Alkalized water - Apple cider vinegar
- Bee pollen - Green juices - Mineral water - Molasses
- Probiotic cultures - Veggie juices - Fresh made juices
- Calcium (pH 12) - Potassium (pH 14) - Sodium (pH 14)
- Magnesium (pH 9) - Cesium (pH 14)
- Baking soda - Lentils - Citrus juices - Olives - Arugula - Cashews

Nutritional Table

Fruit and vegetable nutrional information table							
Food (per 100g)	Calories	Fiber (g)	Sugar (g)	Protein (g)	Fat (g)	Vit-A (IU)	Vit-C (mg)
Apples	52	2.4	10.4	0.26	0.17	54	4.6
Asparagus	20	2.1	1.9	2.2	0.1	756	5.6
Avocado	167	6.8	0.3	2	15.4	147	8.8
Banana	89	2.6	12.2	1.1	0.33	64	8.7
Bell pepper	31	2.1	4.2	1	0.3	3131	128
Blackberry	43	5.3	4.9	1.4	0.5	214	21
Blueberry	57	2.4	10	0.74	0.33	54	10
Broccoli	34	2.6	1.7	2.8	0.4	623	89
Cantaloupe	34	0.9	7.9	0.84	0.2	3382	37
Carrots	41	2.8	4.7	0.9	0.2	16706	5.9
Celery	16	1.6	1.3	0.7	0.2	449	3.1
Cherry	63	2.1	13	1	0.2	64	7
Cranberry	46	4.6	4	0.4	0.1	60	13
Cucumber	15	0.5	1.7	0.7	0.1	105	1.8
Dates	277	6.7	66	1.8	0.2	149	0
Fig	74	3	16	0.8	0.3	142	2
Grapefruit	30	1.1	NA	0.6	0.1	259	37
Grapes	67	0.9	16	0.6	0.4	100	4
Guava	68	5.4	9	3	1	624	228
Kiwi	61	3	9	1.1	0.5	87	93
Lemon	22	0.3	3	0.4	0.2	6	39
Lime	30	2.8	1.7	0.7	0.2	50	29
Mandarin	53	1.8	11	0.8	0.3	681	27
Mango	60	1.6	14	0.8	0.4	1082	36
Olive	115	3.2	0	0.8	11	403	0.9
Onions	40	1.7	4	1.1	0.1	2	7.4
Orange	63	4.5	NA	1.3	0.3	250	71
Papaya	43	1.7	8	0.5	0.3	950	61
Passion Fruit	60	0.2	14	0.7	0.2	943	18
Peach	39	1.5	8	0.9	0.3	326	7
Pear	57	3.1	10	0.4	0.1	25	4.3
Pineapple	50	1.4	10	0.5	0.1	58	48
Plum	46	1.4	10	0.7	0.3	345	9.5
Pomegranate	83	4	14	1.7	1.1	0	10
Potatoes (Baked)	93	2.2	1.2	2.5	0.1	10	10
Strawberry	32	2	5	0.7	0.3	12	59
Tomato	18	1.2	2.6	0.9	0.2	833	14
Watermelon	30	0.4	6.2	0.6	0.2	569	8.1

Information taken from the most recent data from the USDA National Agricultural Library

Quick Healthy Tips

Avoid these foods & ingredients

- **Hydrogenated Oils (or Trans Fats)**
- Oils such as Corn, cottonseed
- **Artificial sweeteners**
    - Aspartame, sucralose
    - sorbitol, maltitol
    - acesulfame K
- High Fructose Corn Syrup or corn syrup
- White sugar
- Processed white flour, white bread
- Sodas (regular or diet)
- **Artificial colors and flavors**
- Hydrolyzed soy protein
- **Monosodium Glutamate (MSG)**
- Don't drink tap water
- Fast food or processed foods
- Deodorants with Aluminum & Paraben
- Instant Oatmeal
- Fried food
- Pork processed meats such as Salami, ham, pepperoni, bacon, etc.

* How to lose weight

- A glass or two of water upon rising
- Eat a big breakfast
- Do a Colon and Liver cleanse
- Don't eat after 7PM
- Eat 5-6 times a day (small portions)
- Eat healthy snacks & fruits twice a day
- Eat green vegetables everyday. They clean the colon
- Drink water (half your weight in ounces each day)
- Walk briskly 45 minutes a day
- No sodas (regular or diet)
- No fast food restaurants
- No high fructose corn syrup
- No processed white flour, white bread
- No artificial sweeteners
- Drink Green Tea every day (2 cups)
- Drink digestive enzymes
- Eat organic grapefruits in the morning
- Fast once or twice a month
- Chew slower when eating

* How to live healthy

- Drink 8 glasses of filtered water/day
- Eat fruits & salads each day
- Eat an apple at least 5 times / week
- Snacks: Walnuts, Almonds, Brazil nuts
- Drink or eat Coral Calcium
- Eat blueberries 3 times per week
- Walk 45 minutes a day
- Breath deeply for 1 minute twice a day
- Drink digestive enzymes (CoQ10, etc.)
- Eat fish (The ones with fins & scales)
- Use Himalayan pink salt
- Eat or drink Flax seed oil & wheat germ
- Eat Omega 3 fatty acids
- Take Vitamins Ester C & E
- Drink Probiotics, Kefir
- Vegetable and chicken soups w/o MSG
- Eat cucumbers, garlic, beans, honey, wheat, barley, olives, avocado
- Do a Colon and Liver cleanse
- No Hydrogenated oils, no sodas, high fructose corn syrup, no fast food, no MSG, no artificial sweeteners & colors

* How to lower Cholesterol

- **Drink Green Tea** every day (2 cups)
- Do a Colon and Liver cleanse
- **Eat an apple & grapes each day**
- **No Hydrogenated Oils (or Trans Fats)**
- Take Cod liver oil
- Drink 8 glasses of filtered water/day
- Drink wheat & Barley grass juice or capsules
- **Eat 2 portions of vegetables and fruits each day** with olive oil and vinegar
- **Walk briskly 35-45 minutes a day**
- Don't smoke
- **Eat fish and less or no red meat**
- **Eat avocados**
- Avoid fried foods
- Reduce sugar consumption
- No sodas (regular or diet)
- Drink Pomegranate juice
- Eat oatmeal cereal Helps to clean the colon
- Take digestive enzymes (CoQ10, etc.)
- Instead of cow's milk, drink almond milk

*These statements have not been evaluated by the FDA and are not intended to diagnose, treat, cure or prevent any disease.

TESTIMONIALS

As a pediatrician my job is not only the diagnosis and management of sick children but the PREVENTION of disease. I feel that prevention should be a priority for pediatricians. I spend most of my time during well visits in discussing safety, upcoming advances and diet. Now, during sick visits, I find myself also trying to prevent disease; not ear infections or sore throat, but diabetes, hypertension and other diseases previously occurring only in adults. All these diseases have one common denominator - OBESITY. In the prevention of obesity lies the key to a long, healthy life. This guide is an easy to read and follow instruction manual on the hidden dangers of food. I have incorporated many of the basic tenets of Mr Aramburo's advice into my daily discussion of a healthy lifestyle. His advice is simple to understand and in its knowledge is the power to prevent "adult" disease from affecting our children, and even in the prevention of disease in ourselves, since parents are the models that children emulate.

Doctora, Monica Florez, MD

Finally a comprehensive and unbiased guide that teaches what we all need to know about the most important nutrients.

Doctor, León Camilo Uribe, MD

Julián, thank you for being such a central person to the major changes I have made in my life when it comes to health and wellness. After being diagnosed with cancer, I was going to blindly follow whatever my doctors were suggesting, which, looking back, was not in my best interest. If it wasn't for you and the information that you gave me that day that we spoke on the phone, I might be dead right now. You opened my eyes to what is really going on in the world, our government, toxicity in our food supply, the dangers of chemo and mammograms, etc. etc. If it wasn't for you I would still be blissfully ignorant. You opened my eyes and my life has never been the same. Though you probably saw our conversation as nothing significant, it was a life-changer for me, and I've made it my mission to educate my friends and family to help them live healthier lives as well. So, THANK YOU, THANK YOU! Your kindness and willingness to share your knowledge had a very large positive impact on my life, my husband's and I am sure, countless others.

Mayte Giubardo Florez, MSW

In 2005 when I started my certifications in Oral Rehabilitation and Cosmetic Dentistry at New York University NYU, I always stopped by West Palm Beach and visited Julian on my way back to my home country Colombia. It was back then when I learned how serious he was about health and the health of others. His willingness to share his knowledge on prevention and healthy eating was eminent and his passion about this subject was clear. That impressed me and every time we talked about this subject during my visits or his visits to Colombia I became more and more interested about healthy eating and living a life style for optimal health. I like to read and do research so I started doing my own research and confirmed everything Julian was telling me including the dangers of certain foods and medicines. After confirming his concerns and learning how to prevent disease I started to change my eating habits and those of my family. I now read the labels before buying any food in the supermarket. In my work with my patients I now share with them the importance of healthy eating and recommend them to always take vitamin C and B complex to maintain good dental and functional health. This has led me to have great success in the treatment of my patients. I trust the tenacity, dedication and seriousness that Julian has gathered through all his research studies. I am pleased and grateful that I have had the opportunity to know him and I congratulate him on this work. I know this book will be an invaluable guide to healthy living for people of all ages. I know this book will give you enough information to live a healthy life and I hope big pharma and big food take notice that consumers are learning more and more about the dangers of processed foods and prescription medications. I also hope these companies make changes for the benefit of the people instead of the pockets of their share holders.

Doctor Jose Heberth Tofiño, Cosmetic Dentistry and Oral Rehabilitation, NYU

I recommend this book for the following reasons: It gives us principles to avoid devastating acute and chronic diseases. It allows us to select healthy foods. It illustrates which foods contain the vitamins we need on a daily basis. It provides comprehensive information on the vital need for water (which in my opinion is the life of the renal system), and water-soluble vitamins and fat. It informs about the need for fiber which in my opinion is the life of the intestines and prevents colon cancer. He offers extensive information on how to prevent diabetes mellitus, heart disease, cancer, Alzheimer's, obesity and the need for the proper PH balance. It teaches us to live healthy, with great recommendations for a healthy diet and daily exercise.

I congratulate Mr. Aramburo because his knowledge and persistent research embodied in this book, gives us vital information and knowledge which are giving me great results in my medical practice with my patients.

Doctor Humberto Delgado Mejía, MD

JUICE AND SMOOTHIE RECIPES

- **Veggie Juice (20 ounces)**
  - 1 medium beet
  - 1 tomatoe
  - 2 carrots
  - 2 red apples
  - 1 cup packed spinach leaves
  - ½ cup parsley
- **Healthy Green Booster (20 ounces)**
  - 1 Granny Smith apple
  - 1 carrot
  - 1 kiwi
  - 1 pear
  - 1 cup packed spinach leaves

- **Super fruit smoothie (25 ounces)**
  - 4 Strawberries
  - 1 banana
  - ¼ cup of blueberries
  - 1 Greek Yogurt, 5 oz
  - 5-6 Blackberries
  - 10 oz spring water
  - 4 oz Orange juice

o **Super Protein (20 ounces)**
- 1 teaspoon of Spirulina
- 1 teaspoon of Chia seeds
- ½ cup blueberries
- 1 Greek yogurt, 5 oz
- 4-5 Blackberries
- 10 oz spring water
- 4 oz orange juice

o **Morning Appetizer (12 ounces)**
- 1 teaspoon of raw almonds
- 1 table spoon of oat meal
- 1 teaspoon of flax seed (ground)
- 5 oz spring water
- 3 oz orange juice
- Half an apple
- 6-7 grapes

o **Natural Detox (12 ounces)**
- 1 Teaspoon of ground flax seed
- 1 Teaspoon of oat meal
- 8 oz of spring water
- 1 orange
- 1 apple
- 1 pear

- **Super Fiber (12 ounces)**
  - 8 oz of spring water
  - Half a banana
  - 7-8 blueberries
  - 7-8 blackberries
  - 6-7 grapes
  - 1 teaspoon oat meal
  - 1 teaspoon Chia seeds
  - 1 teaspoon flax seed

- **Energy Explosion (20 ounces)**
  - 2 celery stocks
  - 1 cup of cranberries
  - 1.5 cups of pineapple cubes
  - Half a banana
  - Half cup spinach
  - 1 teaspoon organic peanut butter
  - 2 table spoons of lemon

- **Healthy reinforcement (20 ounces)**
  - 1 green apple
  - 1 carrot
  - 1 kiwi
  - 1 pear
  - 1 cup spinach
  - Half cup Greek Yogurt
  - 2 table spoons of lemon
  - Half cup crushed ice

- **For the kinds in the morning (20 ounces)**
  - 1 medium apple
  - 2 medium carrots
  - 1 peach without the seed
  - 1 cup of mango chunks
  - 3/4 cup orange juice
  - ½ cup crushed ice
  - Blend and enjoy

- **Healthy Lemonade (8 ounces)**
  - 2 large apples
  - 1 lemon with peel
  - Use juice extractor. Place lemon in between the two apples

- **Berry Medley (16 ounces)**
  - 1 cup frozen mixed berries
  - 11/2 cups almond milk
  - 4 ounces vanilla Greek yogurt
  - ¼ cup of granola

- **Awesome strawberry smoothie (16 ounces)**
  - ½ cup uncooked old fashioned oats
  - 1 cup orange juice
  - 5 ounces vanilla Greek yogurt
  - 4 whole strawberries
  - 1 teaspoon ground flaxseed
  - Crushed ice
  - 1 teaspoon ground cinnamon

- **Banana-Pineapple shake (16 ounces)**
  - 1 cup vanilla Greek Yogurt
  - 4 ounces pineapple cubes or crushed
  - 1 ripe banana
  - 1 teaspoon ground flaxseed
  - 1 cup crushed ice

- **Alkalized water (12 ounces)**
  - 12 ounces spring water
  - 5-6 thin slices of cucumber
    - Let cucumbers infuse the water
  - 10 drops lemon juice
  - 1/5 teaspoon pure baking soda

- **Green and lean smoothie (20 ounces)**
  - 2 cups fresh spinach
  - 1 cup mango chunks
  - 1 cup pineapple cubes
  - ½ banana
  - ½ cup coconut water
  - 1 cup crushed ice

- **Superfoods shake (12 ounces)**
  - 1 cup packed stemmed kale
  - 1 cup baby spinach
  - 1 cup of spring water with crushed ice
  - 1 banana
  - 1 teaspoon Spirulina
  - 1 teaspoon chia seeds
  - 1 table spoon of Green Super Foods powder

REFERENCES

- www.naturalnews.com – Several articles and publications
- Book: Ultra Prevention, Dr Mark Liponis & Mark Hyman
- Book - Ultra Metabolism, Dr Mark Hyman
- Book - The 24 Hour Pharmacist, Suzy Cohen
- Book - A shot in the dark by doctor Harris L Coulter & Barbara Loe Fisher
- Book - Alkalize or Die by doctor Theodore Baroody
- Recipe book Canyon Ranch Cooks by Barry Correia y Scott Uehlein
- Articles from Mayo Clinic, Rochester, Minnesota
- Scientific studies published by the New England Medical Journal
- Scientific studies conducted by Southampton University in England
- Documentary: Fat, Sick and Nearly Dead, Joe Cross, Phil Riverstone, Kurt Engfehr
- Documentary: Forks over Knives, Lee Fulkerson
- Documentary: Food Matters, James Colquhoun, Carlo Ledesma, Andrew Saul, David Wolfe
- Documentary: Food Inc. Robert Kenner
- Documentary: The Beautiful Truth, Charlotte Gerson, Garrett Kroschel, Steve Kroschel
- Documentary: Hungry for Change, James Colquhoun, Laurentine Ten Bosch, Joe Cross, Frank Ferrante

- Documentary: Dying to have known, Stephen Barret, Colin Campbell, Steve Kroschel, Charlotte Gerson
- Documentary: The Gerson Therapy, Max Gerson, Steve Kroschel
- Documentary: Killer at Large, Steven Greenstreet, Bill Clinton, Ralph Nader
- Documentary: Dr Burzinski, the movie. Stanislaw Burzinski.
- The Wall Street Journal, several articles
- The New York Times, several articles
- www.mercola.com Take control of your health
- American Journal of Clinical Nutrition
- World Health Organization website

- Center for Disease Control website
- US Department of Agriculture website
- Environmental Protection Agency website
- Hippocrates Health Institute in West Palm Beach, Florida

ABOUT THE AUTHOR

Mr. Aramburo studied at Florida Atlantic University in Boca Raton, Florida and graduated with a degree in Electrical Engineering. He was born in Colombia, South America and has lived in the West Pam Beach area for over 29 years. He is happily married and has three beautiful children. In the last nine years Julian has been studying and researching multiple books, medical journals and articles on his own related to health and prevention based on proper nutrition.

Julian spends most of his free time reading books on preventive health, reviewing scientific studies, reading general health articles and learning from experts in the alternative medicine field. Healthy living and educating others is his passion and although he doesn't have a degree in medicine or nutrition, his dedication, focus and time spent in this subject has trained him with enough information and education to write this book and dedicate it to his family and close friends. He doesn't consider himself an expert on the subjects covered in this book but he is a good researcher and has a passion for prevention and living a healthy life style.

He loves all kinds of sports including soccer, golf and others but the ones he currently dedicates most of his free time are running and bicycling. He also goes to the gym 4 to 5 times a week and maintains a very active life style. He personally contributes his good health to his exercise routine and his healthy eating habits. He rarely gets sick and when he does he can pin point exactly what has caused his body to be out of balance. When this happens he just puts his body back in balance by eating the right foods (alkaline) and avoiding foods that contribute to poor health (Acid foods).

That's all for now and please don't forget to share this information with your family and close friends so they can also enjoy good health and potentially prevent future diseases. God bless you and your family and please invest in your health today by spending money in prevention rather than medication when you get to your golden years.

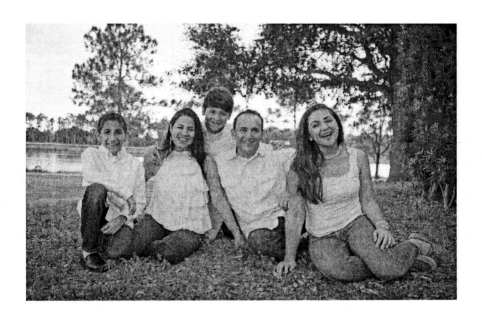